Chinese Medical Gynaecology

A Self-Help Guide to Women's Health

Eddie Dowd

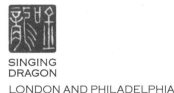

SINGING
DRAGON

LONDON AND PHILADELPHIA

First published in 2018
by Singing Dragon
an imprint of Jessica Kingsley Publishers
73 Collier Street
London N1 9BE, UK
and
400 Market Street, Suite 400
Philadelphia, PA 19106, USA

www.singingdragon.com

Library of Congress Cataloging in Publication Data
Names: Dowd, Eddie, 1972- author.
Title: Chinese medical gynaecology : a self-help guide to women's health /
    Eddie Dowd.
Description: London ; Philadelphia : Jessica Kingsley Publishers, 2018.
Identifiers: LCCN 2017031316 (print) | LCCN 2017042541 (ebook) | ISBN
    9780857013408 (ebook) | ISBN 9781848193826 (alk. paper)
Subjects: LCSH: Gynecology--Handbooks, manuals, etc. | Medicine, Chinese.
Classification: LCC RG111 (ebook) | LCC RG111 .D69 2018 (print) | DDC
    618.1--dc23
LC record available at https://lccn.loc.gov/2017031316

British Library Cataloguing in Publication Data
A CIP catalogue record for this book is available from the British Library

ISBN 978 1 84819 382 6
eISBN 978 0 85701 340 8

Printed and bound in Great Britain

Disclaimer

Every effort has been made to ensure that the information contained in this book is correct, but it should not in any way be substituted for medical advice. Readers should always consult a qualified medical practitioner before undertaking self-treatment. Neither the author nor the publisher takes responsibility for any consequences of any decision made as a result of the information contained in this book.

For more information, please contact Eddie Dowd at: eddiedowd@icloud.com.

Contents

INTRODUCTION

In over a decade of treating gynaecological and obstetrical issues it has become clear to me that Chinese medicine can provide solutions to, and more importantly prevent, many common issues women face on a daily basis.

This book was written to provide information to women who are interested in taking a more active role in their own health and wellbeing. It is not meant as an academic text, and as a result I have only given a very brief synopsis of Chinese medical theory.

Chinese medicine is also completely different to any form of medicine most people will have been exposed to in the past as it makes unique demands on people that biomedicine does not – it will, to some extent, need the patient to make changes in some or all areas of their life.

We, in the West, never think about our health and wellbeing until we get sick, and then we go to the doctor expecting a pill to take away all the symptoms of the illness; as long as the symptoms are gone, we think that the problem has gone away. People in the West have no tradition of seeking to improve their health as they go about their daily lives, and this applies to gynaecology as much as to any other aspect of health.

A question for you – if you, like many other women, suffer from period pain, what do you do about it? Do you take painkillers, go to bed for a couple of days, or just put up with it?

Have you ever thought about what you could do to help yourself? This question can be asked not just about period pain but also a whole host of other gynaecological issues. Of course there are some conditions that are not amenable to self-treatment, but many are, so why not try it?

A VERY BRIEF HISTORY OF CHINESE MEDICINE

The history of Chinese medicine is rooted in the Daoist and Buddhist traditions of China. It originated from the ancient shamanic practices of ancient China and continued to develop out of respect for those principles.

The quintessential texts on the subject of Chinese medicine were first published in the Warring States period (475–221 BC). They detail conversations between the Yellow Emperor (Huang-Di) and six of his advisers at court. The work is composed of two texts, each of 81 chapters, laid out in a question-and-answer format. The first text, the *Suwen* (*Basic Questions*), covers the theoretical foundation of Chinese medicine and its diagnostic methods, while the second, *Ling Shu* (*The Spiritual Pivot*), discusses acupuncture therapy in detail.

From 260 to 265 AD Huang-Fu Mi organised all of the ancient literature into his classic text *Zhenjiu Jia Yi Jing* (*The Systematic Classics of Acupuncture and Moxibustion*). The text is made up of 12 volumes and describes 349 acupuncture points.

Acupuncture developed greatly during the Sui (581–618) and Tang (618–649) Dynasties. On request from the Tang government, the physician Zhen Quan revised the important acupuncture texts and charts. Another famous physician of the time, Sun Si Miao, wrote *Beiji Qian Jin Yao Fang* (*Essential Formulas for Emergencies [Worth] a Thousand Pieces of Gold*). During this period, acupuncture became a special branch of medicine and practitioners were now called acupuncturists. Acupuncture schools appeared and acupuncture education became part of the Imperial Medical Bureau.

During the Song Dynasty (960–1279) Wang Weiyi wrote *The Illustrated Manual on Points for Acupuncture and Moxibustion*. This book accompanied the Bronze Man statue, a life-size model of the acupoints on the human body.

During the Ming Dynasty (1568–1644), classic texts were revised, new techniques and manipulations were developed, and an encyclopaedic work of 120 volumes was written, called *Principles of Acupuncture and Moxibustion*; this was the foundation of the teachings of George Soulié de Morant who introduced acupuncture to Europe.

From 1911 until 1949, Republican China tried to establish a modern state medical system based on Western biomedicine. The practice of traditional medicine was forbidden by the government. However, after the People's Republic of China was formed in 1949, Chinese medicine was re-established as a national system of medicine. China had a huge population and far too few doctors to meet the needs of the people, so Chinese medicine was re-invented and re-introduced to tackle this issue. Chinese medicine was (and still is) able to treat the chronic diseases that were unresponsive to biomedical treatment. By 1955 there were four Chinese medical colleges, and the practice of Chinese medicine became institutionalised nationwide. It now forms part of the state-controlled healthcare system in China.

WHAT IS CHINESE MEDICINE?

Chinese medicine refers to ancient key texts for its theoretical framework, and while biomedicine has a strong scientific basis of anatomy, physiology, biochemistry and molecular biology, Chinese medicine takes a philosophical approach towards the body and maintaining health. Having said that, practitioners of Chinese medicine have always had (and still do) a solid grounding in anatomy (see Chapter 3, for example).

For clarity I have capitalised Chinese medicine terms to distinguish them from biomedicine ones; for example, Heart can be thought of as a functional activity rather than the heart acting as a pump circulating blood.

The basic theory of Chinese medicine is as follows:

- *A holistic ideology:* Humans are part of the universe. Everything within or outside of the body is ultimately interconnected.

- *The Five Vital Substances:* These are fundamental to life and provide the material and functional basis of the body – Qi (Vital Energy or Life Force), Xue (Blood), Jin Ye (Body Fluids), Jing (Essence) and Shen (Spirit/Mind).

- *Yin and Yang theory:* The development of all phenomena in the universe is the result of the interplay of two opposing energies, symbolised by Yin and Yang.

- *Five Element theory:* The Five Elements are seen as existing in a dynamic and balanced relationship with each other. All phenomena and matter in existence are classified in terms of the Five Elements – water, wood, fire, earth and metal.

- *Zang Fu theory:* The concept of 'organ' in Chinese medicine is not equivalent to that in Western medicine. Zang Fu (organs) are better thought of as spheres of functional activity rather than organs in the Western sense of the word.

- *Meridian or Channel theory:* The Meridian system is the system of interconnecting pathways throughout the body in which the Five Vital Substances circulate, connecting all parts of the body into an organic whole.

CHINESE MEDICINE AND GYNAECOLOGY

Within the long history of Chinese medicine there is a history almost as long of practitioners specialising in obstetrics and gynaecology. The first known book on the subject, *Furen Liangfang Jiyao (The Complete Book of Effective Prescriptions for Diseases of Women)*, was published in 1237 AD. It is 24 volumes long and deals with common gynaecological issues, complications of pregnancy and post-partum diseases. As with many classical medical texts much of the information contained within it is still relevant today. Although we now have technology that could never have been imagined when these texts were written, technology doesn't have all the answers, and the ancient and the modern can be combined to yield tangible results, Chinese medicine/IVF (in vitro fertilisation) treatment being a good example. Chinese medicine can be a successful standalone treatment for some common gynaecological conditions, while in other situations it can combine successfully with biomedicine.

Issues that can benefit from either a Chinese medicine or combined Chinese/biomedicine approach include:

- menstrual cycle

- reproductive issues

- pregnancy and post-partum

- menopause

- fertility (especially unexplained infertility)

- fibrocystic breast disease.

DIETARY THERAPY

> **SUN SI MIAO (581–682 AD)** "When treating an illness, the first step should be dietary therapy. Only when this is unsuccessful should you resort to Acupuncture or herbal medicinals."

The concept of food as medicine can be found in all ancient healing traditions, including Greek, Persian, Indian and Chinese medicine. Within some of these traditions the use of food as both a preventive and therapeutic modality has fallen by the wayside in favour of specifically medical or surgical treatment.

Within the sphere of Oriental medicine and Chinese medicine specifically, dietary therapy is still as important a treatment modality as it has always been. Food as medicine is not just a catchphrase; it is a concept that will allow you to begin taking an active role in your own healthcare.

This doesn't necessarily mean that you won't need surgery to remove a fibroid or that you no longer need HRT (hormone replacement therapy) to help deal with menopausal symptoms, but what it does mean is that you will be an active participant in your own healthcare.

The Chinese concept of a balanced diet is very different from that in the West. Chinese medicine takes into consideration not just the nutrient content of foods, such as vitamins and minerals, but also the flavours, the energies and the movements of foods in relation to different body organs.

Eating healthily is not a one-size-fits-all concept; everyone has different needs that will depend on their present state of health, age, occupation, etc. Rather than focusing on weight loss, looking at calories or fat content, Chinese dietary therapy focuses on how food tangibly affects a person. It's not just about weight loss; it's about improving your overall state of health at both a physical and mental level.

The earliest written record of Chinese dietary therapy is Sun Si Miao's *Essential Formulas for Emergencies [Worth] a Thousand Pieces of Gold* (652 AD) in which he discusses the treatment of a variety of diseases through diet; for example, his treatment for goitre included the use of seaweed and the thyroid glands from farm animals. These early iodine and hormone replacement therapies predate Western discoveries by hundreds of years. In 752 AD Wang Shou described his treatment for diabetes. He recommended the use of a pig's pancreas as a treatment, predating the discovery of insulin by a thousand years.

Foods and herbs can have more than one taste or can incorporate all five, and certain tastes are drawn to particular organ systems. As a basic guide:

Salty: Kidneys and Bladder

Sour: Liver and Gall Bladder

Bitter: Heart and Small Intestine

Spicy: Lungs and Large Intestine

Sweet: Spleen and Stomach

The knowledge that certain tastes will affect a specific organ or Channel in a particular way means that food can be used to both prevent and treat specific conditions.

Food can be incredibly powerful medicine just as it can be the cause of a whole host of illnesses. Everyone needs to eat, and so you might as well do so in such a way that enhances your health, not damages it.

In this book I have concentrated on dinner as the 'medicated' meal as so few people have time for breakfast or lunch. The suggestions are generic, but for a personalised plan, talk to a practitioner of Chinese or naturopathic medicine.

Please note that, unless indicated otherwise, all recipes in this book are intended to serve 1–2 people.

Chapter 1

AETIOLOGY AND PATHOLOGY IN CHINESE MEDICINE

WHAT IS AETIOLOGY AND PATHOLOGY?

Aetiology can be looked at as a root cause, which can be physical, mental or emotional in nature.

Pathology is the study of disease. In Chinese medicine pathology is looked at in terms of pattern(s). One disease may have multiple patterns, and multiple patterns may correspond to a single named disease in biomedicine.

Irritable bowel syndrome (IBS) can be used as a practical example of this. In biomedicine IBS is a collection of symptoms with no discernible root cause. In Chinese medicine IBS can be seen in terms of numerous patterns, all requiring different treatment, depending on the root cause. Leaving aside everything except therapeutic outcome, I believe that the search for a root cause to every pathology is what sets Chinese medicine aside from every other medical system.

As most readers of this book will be familiar with Western medicine (biomedicine), we can use that as a comparison. Biomedicine will always seek to identify a particular pathogen, a bacteria or virus, and once identified, the pathogen can be treated. A practitioner of Chinese medicine will always seek the root cause; they will, of course, treat the presenting illness (if appropriate to do so), but they will endeavour to find the reason why the illness manifested in the first place, that is, the root cause. Treating symptoms is only half the treatment. This view is echoed in medical texts from all traditions of Chinese medicine:

Whenever we treat a disease, we must approach it at the base. Base here means root or source. Every stream on earth has a source, and every plant has a root. If all murky sediments settle at the source, the downstream waters will naturally be clear and fresh, and if we water a root, it will grow and branches will sprout; these are the laws of nature. The experienced physician, therefore, will always consider the source. (Zhongzi 1637)

Chinese medicine is a medicine that is deeply rooted in a naturalistic world view where there was, and still is, an awareness that what happens in the macrocosm (universe/the world around us) will be mirrored in the microcosm (the human body).

Contrary to what happened in the West, doctors in China didn't seek to specifically use medical labels for disease patterns; they just applied the theory of macrocosm/microcosm so that diseases are labelled based on which naturally occurring phenomenon has caused them. Classically these pathogenic factors were labelled Wind, Dampness, Dryness, Cold, Heat and Summer Heat. They behave in the human body as they behave in nature. In the West we know that being cold or living in a damp house can cause illness; in Chinese culture and medicine Cold or Damp *are* the illnesses.

Listed below are the environmental pathogens that can cause illness.

Heat and Fire

Heat and Fire are regarded as similar in nature but different in intensity.

Heat and Fire are both Yang-type pathogens that will attack the Yin (cooling, moistening) functions of the body. Thin endometrial lining, lack of cervical mucus (especially at ovulation) and vaginal dryness are all common symptoms of excess Heat.

Damp and Phlegm

Damp is Yin (cool and moist) in its nature and it attacks the body's Yang (moving, active) functions. The presence of fluids in certain body areas is absolutely vital for good health; for example, without synovial fluid in your joints, your body would seize up. It is only when these fluids stagnate or leak into body areas where they shouldn't be that they cause problems.

In specifically gynaecological terms, fibroids are an obvious example of what happens when fluids accumulate and congeal, and most, if not all, the recipes in Chapter 6 on fibroids are focused on draining Dampness.

Dryness

Dryness as a climatic condition tends not to be a big problem in Western Europe, but in its artificial forms it is a major problem. The main artificial forms of dryness are central heating and air conditioning. Dryness is a Yang pathogen that will injure the Yin (cooling and moistening functions) of the body.

Cold

Cold in the body behaves as cold in nature does; it slows the bodily functions down, congeals the flow of fluids and locks things in place. Cold is a Yin pathogen and it will therefore attack the Yang (moving, active) Qi of the body.

If you are one of the many women who find a hot water bottle eases period pain, there is a good chance that Cold lodged with the tissues or Channels of your lower abdomen is the root cause of your issue. A human body is roughly 65 per cent water, so it's not hard to imagine what has happened within the tissues – the cold has turned fluid that is normally free-flowing into a solid mass resulting in stagnation, and stagnation = pain.

EMOTIONAL CAUSES OF DISEASE

Chinese medicine has long recognised that any excessive emotional state has the potential to become pathological and cause physical symptoms. The reason there is no branch of Chinese medicine that deals exclusively with mental or emotional problems is that the mind and body cannot be separated in terms of health or illness.

What is excessive or what could be seen as excessive could cover a broad spectrum. An excess for one individual may be a deficiency for another; for example, some people perform brilliantly under pressure while others crumble.

What constitutes 'excessive' in relation to emotions can be looked at in five ways:

- too much of a particular emotion

- too little of a particular emotion

- the right emotion at the right time but too intense

- an inappropriate expression of emotions

- a complete lack of emotion.

In some cultures a 'grin and bear it' attitude is seen as desirable when dealing with emotional issues, but this only worsens the problem. If a problem is not acknowledged and dealt with, it won't just go away; it will get worse and manifest ever more serious symptoms at all levels. I am personally quite sure that the reason people in certain geographical regions don't seem to suffer with stress-related illnesses (such as heart attacks) is due not only to their diet, but also to their ability to freely express their emotions. The area around the Mediterranean is a good example of this. People in this area eat a diet that is good for their physical health, and they are also not shy about expressing their emotions, which is good for their emotional as well as their physical health.

Practitioners of Chinese medicine will tell you that repressed emotions will cause energetic stagnations at various points in our bodies, and that sooner or later these stagnations will manifest as physical symptoms.

The importance of dealing with the underlying emotional causes of disease cannot be overstated – don't treat just the physical symptoms. This situation can be compared to pulling the flower head off a weed – as any gardener knows, if the root is still there, the weed will grow back.

Stress

It would be impossible to finish this section without discussing stress. If you were to ask a hundred people to define what stress means to them, you would get a hundred different answers as everyone has a different opinion of what stress is.

Stress could be looked at as any sort of strain, either physical, mental or emotional, that is serious enough to upset the proper balance and interactions between any area of the body, mind or spirit. This stress would not necessarily have to reach monumental proportions to become dangerous, as low-grade chronic stress is a major contributing factor in many modern ailments.

CAUSES OF DISEASE THAT ARE NOT INTERNAL/EXTERNAL

This final section covers all factors that don't relate to external pathogens or emotional factors, and includes things such as accidents, animal bites or a car crash. It may seem limiting to just have three, but in reality it's not, as Chinese medicine doesn't treat named conditions but rather patterns of disharmony as they relate to an individual. Everything in these three categories can be put into a diagnostic framework that allows a practitioner to treat any combination of patterns. The apparent simplicity of Chinese medicine is one of its great strengths; the system is so flexible that it can adapt to treat any condition at any level of a person.

REFERENCES AND FURTHER READING

Jingyi, Z. and Xuemei, L. (2012) *Patterns & Practice in Chinese Medicine*. Seattle, WA: Eastland Press.

Johnson, J. A. (2000) *Chinese Medical Qigong Therapy: A Comprehensive Clinical Guide.* Pacific Grove, CA: International Institute of Medical Qigong.

Kaptchuk, T. K. (2000) *Chinese Medicine: The Web that Has No Weaver.* London: Rider, an imprint of Ebury Press, Random House.

Mann, F. (1962) *Acupuncture: The Ancient Chinese Art of Healing and How It Works Scientifically.* London: William Heinemann Medical Books.

Needham, J. (1956) *Science and Civilisation in China, Volume 1.* Cambridge: Cambridge University Press.

Ni, M. (1995) *The Yellow Emperor's Classic of Medicine: A New Translation of the Neijing Suwen with Commentary.* Boston, MA, and London: Shambhala Publications, Inc.

Zhongzi, L. (1637) *Yizong Bidu (A Primer of Medical Objectives).*

Chapter 2

THE FIVE VITAL SUBSTANCES OF CHINESE MEDICINE

Chinese medicine is a complete form of medicine characterised by a unique theoretical system with its own forms of diagnosis, treatment, prognosis and treatment modalities. These originated thousands of years ago through meticulous observation of the interactions between nature, the cosmos and the human body.

Until the middle ages all medicine, Eastern and Western, would have adhered to these naturalistic world views, but with the scientific revolution, a parting of the ways occurred.

Medicine in the Western world adopted the doctrine of specific cause, which postulates that a single micro-organism (bacteria or virus) causes specific illnesses and symptoms, whereas practitioners of Oriental medicine retained their vitalist doctrine, which states that man assists, but nature heals. In biomedicine, disease is something alien to the person, something that must be killed or removed. Treatment tends to be geared towards treating a specific sick organ or fighting an invading bacteria or virus. Chinese medicine treats a person, not a disease. It will, of course, treat symptoms, but the ultimate goal is to find the root cause, to find what makes that person susceptible to that disease, what it is that allows a pathogen to invade or allow an emotional upset to cause a disturbance to the smooth, proper interaction of the various aspects of self. Health is more than the absence of disease.

Gross anatomy (how the body functions) is by far the largest mountain that needs to be climbed before practitioners of the two systems can accept each other, but this understanding may be closer than we think, thanks to work currently being done by physicists and mathematicians. The problem is how we think the world, and human beings as part of that world, work.

Whereas biomedicine takes a structural view of the human system, Chinese medicine emphasises a functional approach. The traditional Chinese view of human physiology is based on the movement of energy, to and from various states of being along defined pathways (Meridians). This movement of energy within is comparable to the concept of energy fields that have arisen in both quantum and contemporary physics. According to this idea, matter and energy (form and function) are inseparable, dependent on each other and defined by each other. The separation of matter and energy, inner and outer, physical and mental is not realistic, as they are the same phenomena viewed from different perspectives:

> ...we are, and are immersed in and are a sea of energy. (Dr Thorsten Ludwig, physicist, 2012)

> We are not onlookers peering into the unified field of separate, objective reality – we are the unified field. We can reach beyond the physical body and extend the influence of intelligence. Every thought you are thinking creates a wave in the unified field. It ripples through all the layers of intellect, mind, senses, and matter, spreading out in wider and wider circles. You are like a light radiating not photons but consciousness. As they radiate, your thoughts have an effect on everything. Your relationship to life is the same as that of one cell to your whole body. One cell can talk to your whole body. One cell can influence your whole body. You can talk to the whole of life – influence the whole of life. The whole of life is as alive as we are. The distinction between 'in here' and 'out there' is a false one – as if the heart disregarded the skin because it was not on the inside. (Deepak Chopra, 2015)

The theory of the Five Vital Substances may seem over-simplistic to the Western mind, but these theories in all their permutations can be successfully applied to any named condition, caused by any pathogen. Language, not the ability to treat illness, is the major barrier here, as many concepts don't translate well, if at all.

The theory presented in this and the following chapters is only a simple synopsis; it can (and does) take a lifetime of study to begin to adequately comprehend it. Always keep in mind that this is a very brief overview of a very complex subject.

THE THEORY OF YIN AND YANG

The concept of Yin and Yang is probably the single most important theory of Chinese medicine, as everything we study and practise is based on this concept.

The principle was formulated in ancient China as a way of explaining all natural phenomena. It is a philosophical concept made from observing the movement of the planets and stars, the rhythmic cycles of seasons and weather, the patterns of day and night, life and death and growth and decay. The ancients realised that polarity (opposites) creates the dynamic field in which Qi (energy) moves, and this movement causes change to occur. This theory was then applied to medicine to explain human physiology and the pathologies that humans can suffer from.

The Chinese character for Yang illustrates the sunny side of the mountain. The character for Yin is drawn as the dark shadow of a mountain.

These characters can be seen as opposites, dark and light or shade and sun, and from this it could also be taken that the day is Yang and the night is Yin.

It was from this observation that a complex system of correspondences developed. The table below is a brief synopsis of this.

Yang	Yin
Above	Below
Bright	Dark
Dryness	Wet
Exterior	Interior
Male	Female
Transformative	Formative
Light	Heavy
Growth	Decay
Intangible	Tangible

It was from these observations that the ancients devised the four laws of opposition, interdependence, consumption and transformation. These laws govern everything within the universe at a macrocosmic level and within the body at a microcosmic level. Although they may appear simple, they are, in reality, extremely complex; for example, the law of opposition says that where there is up there must be down, but where does up end and down begin? This will be totally dependent on a unique situation in a single moment of time.

The four laws that govern Yin and Yang

- *Opposition:* Yin and Yang oppose, balance and complement each other; for example, if there is up there must be down, if there is in there must be out.

- *Interdependence:* One cannot exist without the other. Yin (the organ) requires Yang (Qi) to produce vital substances. There can be no form without function or function without form.

- *Consumption:* When one increases the other decreases. A relative balance is always maintained so that balance (homeostasis) is kept. Yin consumes Yang and Yang consumes Yin in order to survive.

- *Transformation:* Yin can transform to Yang; Yang can transform to Yin and vice versa; for example, day to night and back to day.

The infinite divisibility of Yin and Yang

Yin and Yang are always in a constant state of change; as one waxes the other wanes.

Within Yang there is always some aspect of Yin.

Within Yin there is always some aspect of Yang.

Nothing can ever be truly all encompassing Yin or Yang in nature.

The Taiji symbol

The Taiji (Supreme Ultimate) symbol is known worldwide, and perfectly illustrates the four laws governing Yin and Yang.

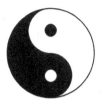

Yin and Yang have their roots in Wuji, an undifferentiated emptiness represented by a circle. This empty circle represents the primordial soup from which everything emerged. Taiji emerges from Wuji and divides the empty circle representing Wuji into Yin and Yang. As Taiji separates right from left, male from female, in from out and Yin from Yang, Taiji is the space where heaven and earth meet, and it forms the boundary between heaven and earth allowing connection and communication but at all times keeping the four laws. Taiji is the potential from which everything that can, does or will exist has emerged.

Yin and Yang as they relate to body areas

Comparable to Western anatomy, Chinese medicine also divides the body into aspects or planes. In Chinese medicine, these classifications are divided into Yin and Yang physical planes and anatomical directions. These divisions assist the practitioner in determining the collection and movement of Qi.

The structural aspects are categorised as follows:

- The cranial or superior aspect (towards the head) of the body's structure is considered Yang; the caudal or inferior portion of the body (towards the feet) is considered Yin.

- The posterior or dorsal portion (back side) of the body is Yang; the anterior or ventral portion (front side) is Yin.

- The superficial aspect (exterior) of the body is Yang; the deep portion (interior) of the body is Yin.

- The left side of the body is Yang; the right side is Yin.

- The lateral aspect (further from the centre) of the body is Yang; the medial portion (middle) is Yin.

- Yin Officials (Zang/solid organs) are considered Yin in nature as they have a storage function.

- Yang Officials (Fu/hollow organs) are considered Yang in nature as their functions are based on transition.

THE FIVE VITAL SUBSTANCES

The Five Vital Substances encompass all substances within the body that are necessary for life to begin and to continue to exist. They all interact with and influence each other in both health and illness. Each manifests in a predictable and specific way; any deviation from this normal expression can be seen as pathological (disease-causing).

Qi (Energy/Potential)

Qi is a fundamental concept in Chinese medicine with multiple levels of meanings. If you read enough in Chinese medicine, you would find that it seems to use Qi to describe almost all invisible forces that affect human life, health and illness. At a basic level this is true – Qi is both the motive force that animates us as well as the glue that binds us at both a microcosmic (body) and macrocosmic (environmental) level. (Please note that there is no adequate English translation of what Qi is or does.)

> **ZHANG ZAI (1020–1077)** "The Great Void consists of Qi and Qi condenses to become the myriad of things. In terms of Chinese medicine Qi is the energetic foundation of the universe, as it is the physical and spiritual substratum of human life."

> **ZHU XI (1131–1200)** "When dispersing Qi makes the Great Void, only regaining its original misty feature, but not perishing; when condensing it becomes the origin of all beings."

Chinese medicine uses the concept of Qi primarily in two senses. The first use is in an abbreviation of function or condition. Qi is used to describe the complex of functional activities of any organ;

for example, Heart Qi is not a refined substance in the Heart, but is both a reflection of and is the Heart's functional activities at all levels (physical, mental, emotional, spiritual and energetic). As you will see, Chinese medicine is more concerned with function rather than form.

The second use of Qi is vital energy, which stems from the Chinese character for Qi. Qi can be decomposed into two radicals that stand for vapour or steam and (uncooked) rice or grain. It is the energy (the potential) within the grain that is called Qi, not the material or chemical part itself. On some levels Qi can be viewed similarly to adenosine triphosphate (ATP), the molecular potential of the energy of biomedicine, but as with many things in Chinese medicine, Qi is assigned a much broader range of functions. It makes sense if you remember that at the time when these theories were developed humans did not have the technology to quantify different aspects of energy. All motive force was called Qi, and where it was active in terms of organs, body areas or Channels defined it, thus the ancients classified 127 types of Qi.

Blood is the mother of Qi and Qi is the commander of Blood.

This statement sums up the relationship between form and function in Chinese medicine. Blood (Yin in nature) nourishes and sustains the Zang and Fu that help produce Qi, while Qi (Yang in nature) provides the motive force and energy to the Zang Fu to produce Blood.

Blood (Xue)

Blood in Chinese medicine is much more than the red fluid that moves within veins and arteries (again, there are issues in translation). In biomedicine blood represents both the intracellular compartment (the fluid inside the blood cells) and the extracellular compartment (the blood plasma).

Put simply, blood carries oxygen and nutrients to the cells while carrying away waste. All this holds true in Chinese medicine. The terminology may be different but the process is essentially the same; however, Blood also carries human conscience within it. Some aspects of your mind/human awareness reside in and are nurtured by the Blood.

This is not a concept that is confined to Chinese medicine. Research conducted by Dr Candace Pert (1999) has conclusively proven that many aspects of what we can regard as human consciousness can be found in the blood. Furthermore, there are numerous reports of recipients of transplanted organs experiencing strange phenomena after surgery, including atypical thoughts, emotions and preferences for foods, lifestyle choices, etc., that are totally uncharacteristic.

The quality of the Blood is an important component of health and fertility in Chinese Medicine theory, and can be interpreted by characteristics of the menstrual flow.

Comparing Qi and Blood

- Blood is a denser form of Qi.

- Blood is inseparable from Qi.

- Qi moves Blood and Blood is the mother of Qi.

- Qi gives life and movement to Blood, but Blood nourishes the organs that produce Qi.

- Blood and Qi flow together in the Channels.

- Blood is the mother of Qi and Qi is the commander of Blood.

This is a basic fact of Chinese medicine. Blood (Yin in nature) nourishes and sustains the Zang and Fu that help produce Qi, while Qi (Yang in nature) provides the motive force and energy to the Zang Fu to produce Blood.

Body Fluids (Jin Ye)

Body Fluids encompasses the full range of fluids within the body except Blood. Mucus, saliva, synovial fluid, etc. can all be subsumed under this heading. The ancients did classify the various types of Body Fluids in terms of their pathological manifestations, but for the purposes of this book, we don't need to worry about these classifications.

This is not to say that Body Fluids are unimportant for the purposes of this book – many common gynaecological issues are rooted in the pathology of Body Fluids; for example, fibroids are often seen and treated as congealed Body Fluids, while at the other end of the spectrum vaginal dryness is often a lack of Body Fluids.

You will notice in many of the recipes in this book that the aim is to drain Dampness (stagnated, congealed fluids) or to build Blood and Body Fluids.

Comparing Body Fluids and Blood

The quote from Mann below shows just how intimately linked Blood and Body Fluids are in Chinese medicine:

> Both Body Fluids and Blood depend on each other intimately, their dependence is totally mutual. Due to their common origin a deficiency of Body Fluid instils a corresponding deficiency of Blood and vice versa. (Mann 1962)

Essence (Jing)

> What life comes from is called Jing. Jing is what the first life impulse comes from. That which precedes the coming into existence of human personality is called Jing. (Ni 1995)

Jing refers to the indispensable bioenergetic substance of all living. It regulates growth and development in the same way as DNA. It could be argued that Jing is comparable to DNA as they have broadly similar functions – the storage of biological information. However, Jing is more than just genetic information; it is a refined essence, the purest, rarest and most concentrated of the Five Vital Substances.

We are all born with a finite amount of Jing, and the very process of living causes a depletion in our reserves, our material foundation, and in women, periods and childbirth accelerate this loss. It is the loss of Jing due to menstruation that causes fertility to decrease so dramatically as a woman ages. It is also why the rate of Down's Syndrome babies born increases from one in 1500 at the age of 25 to one in 32 at age 45. The vital spark that provides the base of primordial substance is weak or in some way compromised as women age. Classical Chinese medical texts made note of the correlation between a woman's age and her ability to conceive, based on the volume of Jing available in the woman.

The following is a quote from *Huangdi Neijing Suwen* (*The Yellow Emperor's Classic of Internal Medicine*):

> In old age, one cannot have children; is that due to the exhaustion of the Jing or is it the fault of the heavenly numbers?

The 'heavenly numbers' refers to the theory that women develop in seven-year cycles (and men in eight-year cycles).

Qi Bo (the Emperor's adviser on medical matters) answers:

In young girls

- At seven years of age, the energy of the Kidneys is plentiful, the milk teeth change, and the hair lengthens.

- At the age two seven ($2 \times 7 = 14$ years) the Ren Mai (Directing Vessel) circulates abundantly, the Chong Mai (Sea of Blood) is prosperous, menses manifests following a determined cycle, the young girl can create (conceive).

- At the age three seven ($3 \times 7 = 21$ years), the energy of the Kidneys is in fullness, the wisdom teeth finish pushing out.

- At the age four seven ($4 \times 7 = 28$ years), the muscles and bones become solid, the hair reaches its greatest length, the body is more robust.

- At the age five seven ($5 \times 7 = 35$ years), the Yang Ming (Stomach) energy begins to weaken, vision to fade, the hair to fall.

- At the age six seven ($6 \times 7 = 42$ years), the energy of the three Yang grow weaker at the top of the body, the face dries out, the hair whitens.

- At the age seven seven ($7 \times 7 = 49$ years), the Ren Mai is empty, the Chong Mai grows weaker, the channels of Earth are obstructed. This is why the body becomes exhausted; the woman is no longer fertile.

Shen (Spirit/Mind)

Like many Chinese words, the meaning of Shen varies depending on the context and characters it is combined with.

The *Huangdi Neijing Suwen* (*The Yellow Emperor's Classic of Internal Medicine*, Simple Questions) states, 'That which cannot be fathomed in terms of Yin and Yang is spirit.'

Shen is used to refer to the outward manifestations of life and activity in the human body. It is used to describe the complexion, the spirit in the eyes, the use of language, responsiveness to questioning and stimulation, posture, vitality and general animation.

REFERENCES AND FURTHER READING

Chen, K. W., Liu, T., Zhang, H. and Lin, Z. (2009) 'An analytical review of the Chinese literature on Qigong therapy for diabetes mellitus.' *The American Journal of Chinese Medicine 37*, 3, 439–457.

Ching, J. (2009) *Mysticism and Kingship in China: The Heart of Chinese Wisdom.* Cambridge: Cambridge University Press.

Chopra, D. (2015) *Quantum Healing: Exploring the Frontiers of Mind/Body Medicine.* London: Penguin/Random House.

Kaptchuk, T. K. (2000) *Chinese Medicine: The Web that Has No Weaver.* London: Rider, an imprint of Ebury Press, Random House.

Mann, F. (1962) *Acupuncture: The Ancient Chinese Art of Healing and How It Works Scientifically.* London: William Heinemann Medical Books.

Needham, J. (1956) *Science and Civilisation in China, Volume 1.* Cambridge: Cambridge University Press.

Ni, M. (1995) *The Yellow Emperor's Classic of Medicine: A New Translation of the Neijing Suwen with Commentary.* Boston, MA, and London: Shambhala Publications, Inc.

Pearsall, P., Schwartz, G. and Russek, L. G. (2000) 'Changes in heart transplant recipients that parallel the personalities of their donors.' *Integrative Medicine: Integrating Conventional and Alternative Medicine 2*, 2, 65–72.

Pert, C. (1999) *Molecules of Emotion.* London: Simon & Schuster.

Sheng, C. (2001) 'Emerging paradigms in mind-body medicine.' *Journal of Alternative and Complementary Medicine 7*, 1, 83–91.

Thorsten, L. (2012) 'Zero Point Energy: The View Point of Modern Physics on the Sea of Energy.' Breakthrough Energy Movement conference, Holland. Available at http://globalbem.com/tag/zero-point-energy

Wang, D. T.-Y. (1992) '"Nei Jing Tu", a Daoist diagram of the internal circulation of man.' *The Journal of the Walters Art Gallery 49/50*, 141–158.

Chapter 3

ORGAN THEORY IN CHINESE MEDICINE

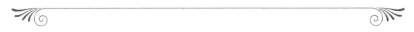

The following quote from Jeremy Ross very succinctly sums up the essence of how Chinese medicine views the internal organs – it is function rather than form that is of importance. This is, of course, not to say that Chinese medicine is ignorant of physical anatomy.

> Chinese medicine has had little interest in anatomical structure; its concern has always been with bodily processes. (Ross 1984)

The earliest historical reference to the dissection of human cadavers is found in *The Book of Han: Annals of Dynastic Literature* (189 BC). The Emperor Wang Mang ordered the dissection of the body of a rebel named Wang Sun Ching. The dissection was performed by the court physician Shang Feng aided by a butcher.

> Measurements were made of the internal organs and bamboo rods were inserted into the blood vessels to discover where they begin and where they end, for the purpose of a better understanding of how to cure disease.

During the Chong Ning period of the Song Dynasty (1102–1106), the bodies of executed bandits were dissected and the findings presented in *Cun Zhen Tu* (*Anatomical Atlas of Truth*).

Chapter 31 of the *Ling Shu* (*Classic of Difficulties* or *The Spiritual Pivot*) is entitled 'Chang Wei' (Stomach and Intestines), and in this chapter the following anatomical measurements are listed:

- Distance from lips to tongue

- Width of the mouth

- Distance from the teeth to the vocal cords (larynx)

- Internal volume of the mouth
- Weight of the tongue
- Length of the tongue
- Weight of the larynx
- Width of the oesophagus
- Length of the oesophagus
- Circumference of the stomach
- Diameter of the stomach
- Maximum capacity of the stomach
- Length of the duodenum jejunum
- Circumference of the small intestine
- Diameter of the small intestine
- Topography of the course of the large intestine
- Circumference of the large intestine
- Diameter of the large intestine
- Length of the gastro intestinal tract from the lips to the anus.

These are only a few examples taken from text books that have been in continuous use for centuries. The reason why I have included this small glimpse at the anatomical knowledge possessed by ancient doctors is to make you aware that although Chinese medicine can seem backwards, with little knowledge of 'scientific medicine', this is simply not the case. The ancients realised that humans were more than physical machines, and Chinese medicine evolved to treat the whole person, not just their physical symptoms.

ZANG FU THEORY

The study of Zang Fu (organs) is the study of the viscera and bowels as they relate to Chinese medicine specifically. Zang or Fu are thought of and studied in terms of functional activity rather than physical form. As you will have seen above, the ancients realised that there was more to a human being than physical form – a human being is a complex mix of physical form, consciousness and emotions, and Zang Fu theory reflects this world view, with every structure in the body viewed as functioning simultaneously on multiple levels. These functions are not based purely on physical anatomy, but also on clinical observation of countless patients over many thousands of years.

In recent decades there have been successive attempts to make the Chinese medical model fit that of biomedicine, and this has led not only to untold confusion, but also to a dilution of Chinese medicine (certainly in the Western world).

I think that Heiner Fruehauf perfectly sums up the problem of trying to make Chinese medicine fit the Western model:

> Since the 18th century, the traditional 'organ' knowledge of Chinese medicine has routinely been compared to the anatomical and biochemical data of the body. However, if we chose to honour the deeper dimensions of Chinese medical theory, the act of training the spotlight of laboratory scrutiny on networks that are primarily energetically defined will look out of place and out of time, quaint to some observers, but outright ridiculous to most. This appears to be the fate of the traditional organ networks. They are increasingly showcased like antiques, quoted in general textbook circumstances but yielding to the parameters of the anatomical organ model in most Chinese medicine clinics in both China and the West. (Fruehauf 2010)

REFERENCES AND FURTHER READING

Davidson, P., Hancock, K., Leung, D. *et al.* (2003) 'Traditional Chinese Medicine and heart disease: What does Western medicine and nursing science know about it?' *European Journal of Cardiovascular Nursing 2*, 3, 171–181.

Fruehauf, H. (1999) 'Chinese Medicine in Crisis: Science, Politics and the Making of "TCM".' *The Journal of Chinese Medicine, October 1999.*

Johnson, J. A. (2000) *Chinese Medical Qigong Therapy: A Comprehensive Clinical Guide.* Pacific Grove, CA: International Institute of Medical Qigong.

Kaptchuk, T. K. (2000) *Chinese Medicine: The Web that Has No Weaver.* London: Rider, an imprint of Ebury Press, Random House.

Needham, J. (1979) *The Grand Titration: Science and Society in East and West.* Boston, MA: Allen & Unwin.

O'Brien, K. A. and Xue, C. C. L. (2003) *A Comprehensive Guide to Chinese Medicine.* River Edge, NJ: World Scientific Publishing Co.

Ross, J. (1984) *Zang Fu: The Organ Systems of Traditional Chinese Medicine.* Edinburgh: Churchill Livingstone.

Zhang, Y. H. and Rose, K. (2001) *A Brief History of Qi.* Brookline, MA: Paradigm Publications.

Chapter 4

CHANNEL (MERIDIAN) THEORY

> **LIU YANCHI (BEIJING COLLEGE OF TRADITIONAL CHINESE MEDICINE)** "The channels of Chinese medicine are not analogous to any tangible channel in the human body, such as the veins and arteries. Rather, they are a way of describing the flow of Blood, Qi, and information that supports the life functions of the body."

A NOTE ON TRANSLATION

'Meridian' is an English reproduction of the French *méridien*, used by George Soulié de Morant for the term *mài* in his translation of the *Huangdi Neijing* (*The Yellow Emperor's Classic of Internal Medicine*). I have used the term 'Channel' throughout this book as I think it is a better, more literal, translation.

CHANNEL THEORY

The Channel systems were first presented in the *Huangdi Neijing* (*The Yellow Emperor's Classic of Internal Medicine*), compiled during the Han Dynasty (206–220 AD). It begins with a mission statement: 'To preserve and protect acupuncture, so it won't be forgotten, obliterated and lost.'

After the Communist revolution in China in the late 1940s and early 1950s, how acupuncture was taught and practised changed drastically. Much of the ancient knowledge found in classical medical texts was cast aside in favour of what many practitioners of classical Chinese medicine now refer to as herbalised acupuncture (a description first used by Ted Kaptchuk in the mid-1980s).

Twelve Channels that are viewed as extensions of the internal organs (Zang Fu) are used to treat pathological patterns. These 12 'Primary' Channels have become the standard for modern acupuncture treatment, while study of the 'Secondary' or 'Divergent' Channels is rare in acupuncture colleges today.

In classical acupuncture, treatment is based on the Channels themselves, as in pathology the Channels represent stages within the pathological process.

THE 12 PRIMARY CHANNELS

The 12 Primary Channels cover the body bilaterally, one on each arm and one on each leg. Each Channel has its individual regular course with a deep internal and a more superficial external pathway. The superficial external pathway is the portion of the Channel that contains acupuncture points, and by stimulating points on the exterior of the body, you can influence structures deep inside the body.

CONNECTING VESSELS

The Connecting Vessels can be divided into major connections as well as into many smaller and more superficial connections. These form a network spanning the entire body – there is nowhere that does not receive Qi and Blood.

DIVERGENT MERIDIANS (CHANNELS)

The 12 Divergent Meridians are branches off the 12 Primary Channels and share the function of circulating Qi throughout the body. The energetic field of the 12 Divergent Meridians forms an enormous web of complex interconnections within the body's 12 Primary Channels.

One of the primary functions of the Divergent Meridians is to integrate all parts of the body with the 12 Primary Channels. There are areas in the body that are not traversed by the pathways of the 12 Primary Channels, as well as organs that are otherwise unconnected, or only remotely connected, by the Primary Meridians.

SINEW CHANNELS

The Sinew Channels flow within the muscles, tendons, ligaments and between the layers of fascia (connective tissue). They bind the bones and allow for joint movement and muscle flexion. Issues of physical structure are typically treated via these.

EIGHT EXTRAORDINARY CHANNELS (MERIDIANS)

These eight Extraordinary Channels are different to the standard 12 Primary Channels in that they are considered to be storage vessels or reservoirs of the Five Vital Substances, and are not associated directly with the Zang or Fu (organs).

REFERENCES AND FURTHER READING

Flaws, B. (Translator) (1999) *The Classic of Difficulties: A Translation of the Nan Jing.* Boulder, CO: Blue Poppy Press.

Jarrett, L. S. (1999) *Nourishing Destiny: The Inner Tradition of Chinese Medicine.* Richmond, MA: Spirit Path Press.

Kaptchuk, T. K. (2000) *Chinese Medicine: The Web that Has No Weaver.* London: Rider, an imprint of Ebury Press, Random House.

Larre, C. and Firebrace, P. (1996) *The Way of Heaven: Neijing Suwen Chapters 1 & 2.* London: Monkey Press.

Larre, C., Rochat de la Vallee, S. J. and Rochat de la Vallee, E. (1995) *Rooted in Spirit: The Heart of Chinese Medicine.* New York: Barrytown/Station Hill.

Ni, M. (1995) *The Yellow Emperor's Classic of Medicine: A New Translation of the Neijing Suwen with Commentary.* Boston, MA, and London: Shambhala Publications, Inc.

Ross, J. (1984) *Zang Fu: The Organ Systems of Traditional Chinese Medicine.* Edinburgh: Churchill Livingstone.

Wieger, L. (1965) *Chinese Characters: Their Origin, Etymology, History, Classification, and Signification. A Thorough Study from Chinese Documents.* New York: Dover Publications.

Chapter 5

ENDOMETRIOSIS

ENDOMETRIOSIS IN BIOMEDICINE

The root cause of endometriosis is unknown in Western medicine, and as a syndrome it was only recognised for the first time in the 1920s. While the true prevalence of endometriosis worldwide is unknown, it is estimated to occur in 10 per cent of women of reproductive age and is present in up to 60 per cent of women who present in clinics with period pain as their primary complaint.

Endometriosis is a difficult condition to diagnose because the symptoms that are experienced are not unique to it. Truly reliable, non-invasive procedures for diagnosis of this disease are lacking, and currently the most common method of diagnosis is by laparoscopic visual inspection (a fibre optic camera inserted into the abdomen where a surgeon can see the lesions).

There are five common theories as to what causes endometriosis:

- Menstrual blood flows backwards through the fallopian tube into the abdominal cavity, where the tissue implants and grows in response to monthly hormonal changes, causing internal bleeding that leads to endometrial lesions.

- Lymphatic dissemination: Endometrial cells pass into the lymph glands and migrate to other areas of the body where they react to monthly hormonal changes.

- Coelomic metaplasia theory: The cells of the endometrium and peritoneum share a common origin in the coelomic endothelium. Inflammation may cause peritoneal cells to transform into endometrial cells, thus causing endometriosis.

- Immune theory: Endometriosis is an autoimmune condition and the symptoms are the result of a hypersensitive immune system attacking itself.

- Genetic factors: A familial tendency to develop the disease has been noted among some researchers.

COMMON SYMPTOMS

The severity of endometriosis is graded from Grade 1 (least severe) to Grade 4 (most severe) according to the amount of endometrial tissue and adhesions found on investigation. In reality the amount of pain a woman feels correlates very little with the extent of her endometriosis; some women have little or no pain despite having extensive endometriosis, while others may have severe pain even though they only have a few small areas of endometriosis. Pain is the major symptom. Typically this is in the lower abdominal, lower back or pelvic regions.

Common symptoms of endometriosis-related pain are as follows:

- Period pain (dysmenorrhoea). This is often the symptom that causes the investigation that leads to a diagnosis of endometriosis.

- Chronic pelvic pain, typically accompanied by lower abdominal pain.

- Urinary urgency, frequency and possibly pain on passing urine (dysuria).

- Painful sex (dyspareunia). This is a common symptom.

- Rectal pain (proctalgia). This pain may occur at any time, but the most common triggers seem to be bowel movements or hormonal changes around ovulation or menstruation.

- Inflammation. The lesions caused by endometriosis react to hormonal stimulation and break up or bleed at the time of a period. This blood accumulates locally, causing inflammation. Over time adhesions (internal scar tissue) can develop and bind internal organs such as the fallopian tubes, ovaries, uterus, bowels and the bladder to each other.

- Chronic pain. In some cases endometriotic lesions can develop their own nerve supply, creating a direct and two-way interaction between the lesions and the central nervous system. In these cases there is often a more or less constant pelvic or abdominal pain that is unrelated to the menstrual cycle. However, pain levels can increase at the time of a period as endometrial lesions elsewhere in the pelvis or abdomen respond to hormonal stimulation and begin to break down.

- Sub-fertility. Many women who have issues conceiving have endometriosis. It is easy to assume that the anatomical distortions and adhesions caused by endometriosis will cause compromised fertility, but in practice there is often no clear link between endometriosis and sub-fertility (from a Western medicine point of view).

ENDOMETRIOSIS IN CHINESE MEDICINE

The earliest mention of the term 'blood stasis' (Xue Dao; literally, uterus-related diseases) can be found in Chapter 75 of the *Huangdi Neijing* (*The Yellow Emperor's Classic of Internal Medicine*). Endometriosis was not recorded in any of the classical Chinese medical texts as a defined entity, but the symptoms are, and always have been, treated under the categories of dysmenorrhoea, irregular menstruation, abdominal mass and infertility.

In his book *The Genius of China: 3,000 Years of Science, Discovery, and Invention*, a popular distillation of Joseph Needham and his collaborators, Robert Temple states:

In China, indisputable and voluminous textual evidence exists to prove that the circulation of the blood was an established doctrine by the second BC at the latest. For the idea to have become elaborated by this time, however, into the full and complex doctrine that appears in The Yellow Emperor's Manual of Corporeal Medicine (China's equivalent of the Hippocratic writings of Greece), the original notion must have appeared a very long time previously. It is safe to say that the idea occurred in China about two thousand years before it found acceptance in the West. (Temple 2007)

Endometriosis results from the stagnation of Blood flow in the pelvis and abdominal regions. The Liver, Spleen and Kidney Channels all run through the pelvis and lower abdomen, and if any of these is blocked, congested or deficient, this will usually manifest in women as some sort of menstrual problem (see the 'Channel theory' section in Chapter 4).

DIETARY CONSIDERATIONS

Trans fats

Most Western diets contain too many trans fats (the fat found in processed food), and many medical practitioners feel these are the root cause of chronic inflammation, including that typically occurring with endometriosis.

Trans fats block the production of type 1 and 3 prostaglandins, which are derived from omega-3 and 6 fats. These fight inflammation (as well as benefiting the hormonal system). Trans fats don't, however, block the production of type 2 prostaglandins that increase inflammation.

An article by Stacey A. Missmer, published in *Human Reproduction*, confirms this link between trans fats and endometriosis. Missmer studied 12 years of data from the Nurses' Health Study II (a total of 70,709 women contributed 586,153 person-years of data):

> ...1199 cases of laparoscopically confirmed endometriosis were reported. Although total fat consumption was not associated with endometriosis risk, those women in the highest fifth of longchain omega-3 fatty acid consumption were 22% less likely to be diagnosed with endometriosis compared with those with the lowest fifth of intake. In addition, those in the highest quintile of trans-unsaturated fat intake were 48% more likely to be diagnosed with endometriosis. (Missmer 2010)

The most likely explanation for this is that trans fats increase circulating levels of several inflammatory markers. These affect other tissue as well, for example those in your bowel or heart, so trans fats are bad all round.

Prostaglandins

Prostaglandins are a group of compounds that have diverse hormone-like effects in animals, including humans. They are made at the sites of tissue damage and control processes such as inflammation, blood flow, the formation of blood clots and the induction of labour. Prostaglandins break down into three different forms: E1 (PGE1), E2 (PGE2) and F2a (PGF2a). While PGE1 can help alleviate endometriosis symptoms, PGE2 causes pain and PGF2a can cause vomiting, nausea and diarrhoea.

The goal of a controlled diet is to reduce the amount of inflammatory prostaglandins in your system, and by changing your diet, it is possible to block PGE2 and PGF2a while encouraging the production of PGE1 to help symptoms. One of the easiest ways of doing this is by changing the types of oils that are taken into your diet. These oils are composed of omega-3 fatty acids, which lead to positive prostaglandin production. Good sources of omega-3 fatty acids include tofu, walnuts, flaxseeds/oil and chia seeds.

It is also important to decrease your intake of those fatty acids that will stimulate an inflammatory response. These are commonly found in saturated fats, butter, animal and organ meat as well as lard. In short, your diet should largely consist of vegetables, nuts, fruit and fish, with very little red meat. This doesn't mean that you can never eat a steak again (assuming you want to), however; as with most dietary restrictions, once the symptoms cease, you can reintroduce animal products. Most women will find a level of saturated fat that they can tolerate without aggravating their endometriosis.

Prostaglandins and non-steroidal anti-inflammatory drugs (NSAIDs)

NSAIDs work by blocking all prostaglandin production. If your period pain or any other symptoms of endometriosis are lessened by taking NSAIDs such as aspirin or ibuprofen, try taking a high-quality cold-pressed omega-3 supplement and see what it does for your pain levels.

Fibre

A diet high in fibre can decrease total circulating oestrogens and xenoestrogen; this should help relieve much of the pain associated with endometriosis.

VITAMIN AND MINERAL SUPPLEMENTS

For a full listing of the actions of common supplements according to Chinese medical theory, see Appendix B.

Although the best source of vitamins and minerals is through a well-balanced diet, many foods today are lacking in these vital trace elements. A point I always try and stress to people is that cheap supplements are cheap for a reason. Discount supplements often use raw ingredients that are low quality and have a poor level of absorption.

The following supplements may be of use in treating the symptoms of endometriosis:

Vitamin A: Helps thin blood and reduces clotting.

B vitamins: Reported to improve the emotional symptoms of endometriosis, and have proved helpful in dealing with premenstrual tension (PMT). Take a B complex rather than individual B vitamins.

Vitamin C: Well known for helping to boost the immune system and providing resistance to disease. It is also used in the body to build and maintain collagen.

Vitamin E: Plays an important role by increasing oxygen-carrying capacities and also strengthens the immune system.

Calcium: Levels of calcium in menstruating women decrease 10 to 14 days before the onset of menstruation. Deficiency may lead to muscle cramps, headache or pelvic pain. Take a supplement that combines calcium and magnesium as they work in tandem.

Iron: Women with endometriosis tend to have very heavy periods that can lead to iron deficiency. This can lead to anaemia, which is characterised by extreme fatigue and weakness.

Magnesium: Can help stop muscle cramps and spasm.

Selenium: When taken together with vitamin E, this has been reported to decrease inflammation associated with endometriosis.

Zinc: Essential for normal enzyme activity within the body. If you are deficient in zinc, it is highly likely that you are suffering from hormonal imbalances.

THERAPEUTIC RECIPES

For a complete listing of the energetic qualities and uses in Chinese medicine of most common foods, see Appendix A.

Breakfast

Porridge made with water and sprinkled with cinnamon. Porridge is warming in nature; it improves digestive function and Blood circulation. Cinnamon improves Blood circulation in the smaller vessels such as those in the fingers, toes or around the reproductive organs.

Walnuts and/or cashews in natural yoghurt. Although yoghurt is considered cold in nature, both walnuts and cashews are warming. It is important to choose yoghurt with no added sugar and with live bacteria.

Lunch

Salad: Many salad vegetables are cold in nature (this can slow down digestive function and impair the movement of Qi and Blood), but the addition of onions, garlic, ginger, chilli or peppers can mediate the cooling action of the vegetables.

Try some of the following combinations:

Carrot, apple and ginger

Carrot and radish

Duck, watercress and orange

Guacamole

Mixed beans with chilli

Prawns with bean sprouts

Dinner

STIR-FRIED NOODLES WITH ASPARAGUS

Ingredients

- 100 g (3½ oz) fresh rice noodles
- 60 g (2 oz) asparagus, trimmed and cut into 5 cm (2 inch) slices
- 2 tsp toasted sesame oil
- 2 cloves garlic, crushed
- 2 cm (⅘ inch) fresh root ginger, grated or finely chopped
- 2 tbsp rice wine (or sherry)
- 2 tbsp soy sauce
- 1 tbsp miso paste
- 2 tbsp sesame seeds, toasted
- black pepper

Method

1. Cook the noodles in plenty of boiling, salted water until tender, and keep warm.

2. Add the asparagus and sesame oil to a frying pan or wok, and cook over a medium heat until tender.

3. Add the garlic, ginger, rice wine, soy sauce and miso paste, stirring for a couple of minutes.

4. Sprinkle with the toasted sesame seeds, season and serve.

Therapeutic qualities

Asparagus: Clears Heat and promotes Blood circulation.

Miso: Promotes the proper movement of urine and tonifies Qi.

Black pepper, garlic and ginger: Warming in nature and move stagnant Blood.

Sesame seeds and oil: Act as an envoy, guiding the actions of the other ingredients to their target organs (Kidneys and Liver).

Rice noodles and soy sauce: Clear Empty Heat and reduce swelling.

Rice wine: Moves Qi and Blood, and thus stops pain.

 ## VEGETABLE AND NOODLE STIR FRY

Ingredients

- 100 g (3½ oz) fresh rice noodles
- 1 medium head pak choi (bok choy) (or cabbage), cut into strips
- 1 tbsp sesame oil
- 6 shiitake mushrooms, sliced
- 2 cm (⅘ inch) fresh root ginger, grated or finely chopped
- 2 cloves garlic, grated or finely chopped
- 1 whole dried red chilli, seeded and finely sliced
- 1 tbsp rice wine (or sherry)
- 1 tbsp soy sauce
- 1 tbsp balsamic vinegar
- 2 tbsp toasted sesame oil
- 1 spring onion (scallion), finely sliced
- 2 tbsp sesame seeds, toasted
- black pepper

Method

1. Cook the noodles in plenty of boiling, salted water until tender, and keep warm.

2. Steam the pak choi, and keep warm.

3. Heat the sesame oil in a frying pan or wok, and fry the shiitake mushrooms, ginger, garlic, chilli, rice wine and soy sauce until fragrant (about 30 seconds).

4. Add the cooked noodles and pak choi.

5. Mix in the balsamic vinegar and toasted sesame oil, and garnish with the spring onion and toasted sesame seeds. Season and serve.

Therapeutic qualities

Shiitake mushrooms: Well known as a stimulant that improves Qi and Blood circulation. Biomedical research shows that a compound within shiitake mushrooms (lentinan) inhibits the production of cancerous cells, and this is already being used by the Japanese pharmaceutical company Ajinomoto to treat stomach cancers. If the autoimmune theory of what causes endometriosis is correct, the cure may lie in medicinal mushrooms.

Garlic, chilli, ginger and spring onion: All have blood-thinning and blood-moving qualities.

Rice noodles and soy sauce: Clear Empty Heat and reduce swelling.

Pak choi: Clears any stagnant Heat via the Intestines.

Sesame seeds and oil: Act as an envoy, guiding the actions of the other ingredients to their target organs (Kidneys and Liver; see Chapter 3).

 PINEAPPLE CURRY

Ingredients

- 1 tbsp curry paste (see below)
- 2 cloves garlic, unpeeled
- olive oil
- 500 g (1 lb) pineapple, diced
- 60 g (2 oz) sweetcorn
- 10 mushrooms (button mushrooms work well)
- ½ onion, finely sliced
- 1 tsp dried thyme
- ½ tsp paprika
- sea salt
- 1 tbsp soy sauce
- 2 tsp cornflour (cornstarch)

CURRY PASTE

- 20 ml (½ fl oz) sunflower oil
- 1 red chilli, deseeded and finely chopped
- 1 clove garlic, grated or finely chopped
- 2 cm (⅘ inch) fresh root ginger, grated or finely chopped

- 1 tsp ground cumin
- 1 tsp ground coriander
- 1 tsp ground black pepper
- 1 tsp fennel seeds
- 1 tsp mustard seeds
- 1 tsp ground turmeric
- 1 tsp ground cinnamon

Method

1. Blend all the ingredients for the curry paste, and set aside.

2. Drizzle the garlic cloves with a little olive oil, wrap in foil and roast at 190°C/Gas Mark 5/375°F for 15 minutes. Once cooked, squeeze out the garlic paste and set aside.

3. Heat the olive oil in a large pan over a medium heat, add the pineapple, sweetcorn, mushrooms, onion, curry paste, thyme, paprika, sea salt, soy sauce and roasted garlic paste, and cook for 10 minutes.

4. Meanwhile, in a small bowl, combine the cornflour with a little water, and stir to make a smooth paste.

5. Reduce the heat to low and add the cornflour mix to the pan. Stir constantly until thickened. Serve.

Therapeutic qualities

Pineapple: Clears Empty Heat and builds Body Fluids.

Sweetcorn: Promotes urination and clears Heat.

Mushrooms: Clear Toxic Heat and nourish the Kidneys.

Soy sauce: Clears Empty Heat.

SALMON CURRY

Ingredients

- 1 tsp cornflour (cornstarch)
- 1 tsp curry powder
- 150 g (5 oz) salmon fillet, cut into thick strips
- sesame oil
- ½ small onion, halved and sliced lengthways
- 1 tsp fresh root ginger, grated or finely chopped
- 1 tsp garlic, grated or finely chopped
- sea salt
- 60 ml (2 fl oz) chicken, fish or vegetable stock
- 1 tbsp curry paste (see above)
- ½ green pepper (bell pepper), cut into strips
- ½ red pepper (bell pepper), cut into strips

Method

1. Combine the cornflour and curry powder with water, and mix to make a smooth paste.

2. Place the salmon strips in a bowl. Add half of the cornflour and curry powder mixture and coat the salmon.

3. Heat the sesame oil in a wok or frying pan and fry the salmon for a few minutes on each side, until golden brown. Drain the oil and discard.

4. Add more sesame oil to the frying pan or wok and fry the onion, ginger and garlic (about 30 seconds).

5. Add the sea salt, stock, curry paste and remaining cornflour and curry powder mixture, and mix well. Toss in the peppers and stir-fry for 1 minute. Add the salmon strips and toss gently to coat with the sauce. Serve.

Therapeutic qualities

Salmon: Nourishes Blood and Yin.

Green and red peppers: Promote Blood circulation and reduce swelling.

Ginger and garlic: Move Blood and help relieve pain.

Curry paste: Moves Blood and helps relieve pain.

SALMON AND GINGER FISHCAKES

Ingredients

- 140 g (5 oz) salmon fillet, finely chopped
- 2 tsp fresh root ginger, grated or finely chopped
- zest of 1 small lime
- black pepper and sea salt
- 1 tsp sesame oil

Method

1. Mix the salmon in a bowl with the ginger, lime zest and seasoning.
2. Chill before forming small patties.
3. Heat the sesame oil in a frying pan and cook the patties for 3–4 minutes each side, until golden brown and cooked through. Serve.

Therapeutic qualities

Salmon: Nourishes Yin and helps prevent inflammation.

Ginger: Moves Blood and prevents Blood stasis.

Lime zest: Moves Qi and harmonises the digestive system. Its aromatic nature prevents the oily salmon becoming cloying and damp.

Sesame oil: Moves Qi and Blood.

GINGER AND CRAB WITH SPRING ONIONS

Ingredients

- 1 crab, cooked (about 680–900 g or 1½–2 lbs)
- 3 tbsp cornflour (cornstarch)
- oil for deep frying
- 1 tbsp sesame oil
- 5 cm (2 inches) fresh root ginger, grated or finely chopped
- 3 spring onions (scallions), cut into 5 cm (2 inch) lengths

SAUCE

- 1 tbsp oyster sauce
- 1 tsp ground white pepper
- 1 tsp sesame oil
- 2 tsp brown sugar
- 6 tbsp water
- 4 tsp cornflour (cornstarch)
- 1 tsp fish sauce

Method

1. Combine all the ingredients for the sauce in a bowl, and set aside.
2. Cut the cooked crab into pieces. Place in a bowl.
3. Add the cornflour to the bowl and lightly coat the crab pieces with it.
4. Heat the oil in a wok or frying pan. When the oil is hot, drop the crab pieces in and deep fry. As soon as they turn red, remove them, strain off any excess oil and set aside.
5. Add the sesame oil and ginger to the wok or frying pan and stir-fry until aromatic. Add the crab pieces and stir-fry to warm through before adding the sauce.
6. Add the chopped spring onions, toss the crab around in the wok a few times until well coated with the sauce, and serve.

Therapeutic qualities

Crab: Breaks Blood stasis. Crab is so effective at dissipating congealed Blood that women in the early stages of pregnancy are advised not to consume it (as a foetus at this stage is basically just a sack of blood cells).

Ginger, spring onions and white pepper: Are all aromatic and warm in nature. They counteract the extreme cold nature of the crab, as well as moving Qi and Blood (improving micro-circulation). Their aromatic nature prevents the sugar becoming cloying.

Brown sugar: Its warm, sweet nature harmonises the digestive system. As the cold nature of the crab can slow down the digestive process, the brown sugar counteracts this.

Sesame oil: Moves Qi and Blood.

PRAWN STIR FRY

Ingredients

- 2 tbsp olive oil
- 2.5 cm (1 inch) fresh root ginger, grated or finely chopped
- 2 garlic cloves, grated or finely chopped
- 1 tsp chilli flakes
- 100 g (3½ oz) raw king prawns
- 80 g (3 oz) broccoli, trimmed into florets
- 80 g (3 oz) mange tout, sliced into pieces
- 1 tbsp sweet chilli sauce
- juice of half a lime
- handful of fresh coriander leaves (cilantro)
- handful of toasted cashew nuts

Method

1. Heat the olive oil in a frying pan or wok over a high heat and stir-fry the ginger, garlic and chilli flakes for a couple of minutes, then add the prawns and cook for 2–3 minutes until pink. Remove from the pan and set aside.

2. Add the broccoli florets to the pan with a splash of water and cook for 2–3 minutes, then add the mange tout and stir in the sweet chilli sauce, lime juice and coriander leaves.

3. Return the prawns to the pan, mix well, then sprinkle with the toasted cashew nuts and serve.

Therapeutic qualities

Cashew nuts: Tonify Kidney Qi. The Kidneys contribute in large part to reproductive function.

Prawns: Are very hot in nature; they strongly tonify Kidney Qi and improve Blood circulation.

Broccoli: Tonifies Blood. The cool nature of broccoli and mange tout help balance the dish with so many other ingredients of a warm or hot nature included.

Mange tout: Harmonises the digestive system.

Garlic, ginger and chilli: All move Qi and Blood (improve micro-circulation).

Lime juice: Acts as an astringent and prevents reckless movement (over-stimulation) of Blood by the hotter ingredients in the recipe.

ACUPRESSURE

How to apply pressure to the points

To press points, use something blunt. You can use finger pressure, but if you have to apply sustained pressure, you may find it uncomfortable. A chopstick (like the ones you get with a takeaway meal) is ideal for this purpose.

Ideally have someone do the treatment for you; that way you are not creating muscular tension while you try and reach points. You can also focus more on what sensations (or lack of them) result from pressing the point.

Don't press too hard; use enough pressure that you (or your partner) can feel something happening.

When you get to the point where something is happening, keep the pressure constant and hold for 30 seconds.

If you are not feeling any effects from pressing a point, you may not be pressing on the exact right spot. Try different spots around the location you first tried.

The points

Any number of points can be used, and in most cases points used in an acupuncture treatment are selected based on signs and symptoms presenting at that time. The points listed below are all useful in the treatment of endometriosis, but for a more individualised treatment plan, talk to a licensed acupuncture practitioner.

LIVER 5 (LI GOU) WOODWORM CANAL

Actions – Regulates Qi, benefits the genitals, clears Dampness and Heat from the pelvic region and regulates menstruation.

Location – Five finger breadths above the tip of the medial malleolus on the midline of the medial surface of the tibia.

Location note – Follow the bone on the inside of your leg upward for five finger breadths.

LIVER 9 (YIN BAO) YIN BLADDER

Actions – Adjusts menstruation and regulates the pelvic region.

Location – Four finger breadths above the medial epicondyle of the femur between the vastus medialis and sartorius muscles.

Location note – Start from the top of the bone on the inside edge of your knee, four finger breadths up (towards the groin) where there is a tender spot in the muscle.

LIVER 11 (YIN LIAN) YIN CORNER

Actions – Benefits the uterus.

Location – Two finger breadths directly below the lateral border of the pubic bone at the proximal end of the thigh below the pubic tubercle and on the lateral border of the abductor longus muscle.

Location note – Find the edge of your pubic bone and drop straight down two finger breadths.

STOMACH 31 (BI GUAN) THIGH GATE

Actions – Promotes Qi and Blood circulation in the pelvis and legs.

Location – On the upper thigh, in a depression just lateral to the sartorius muscle at the junction of a vertical line drawn downward from the anterior superior iliac spine and a horizontal line drawn level with the lower border of the pubic symphysis.

Location note – The point is lateral (to the outside) to Liver 11 (Yin Lian).

STOMACH 36 (ZU SAN LI) LEG THREE LI

Actions – Tonifies Qi and nourishes Blood; calms the mind.

Location – Three finger breadths below the lower border of the kneecap and one finger breadth from the anterior border of the tibia (shin bone).

LARGE INTESTINE 4 (HE GU) PEACEFUL VALLEY

Actions – Alleviates pain.

Location – On the dorsum of the hand between the first and second metacarpal bones, approximately in the middle of the second metacarpal bone on the radial side.

Location note – Between the thumb and first finger, just above the web.

Caution – This point can induce labour, so do not use if pregnant.

REN 4 (GUAN YUAN) ORIGIN PASS

Actions – Tonifies the Kidneys, benefits the uterus and assists conception.

Location – Three finger breadths straight down from your belly button.

ADJUNCT SELF-TREATMENTS
Femoral massage

This massage increases the blood flow to the pelvic organs. This increased blood flow may be useful in clearing any stagnations in the pelvic region (many acupuncture or herbal treatments will be trying to accomplish the same thing, albeit a bit more forcefully).

Locating your femoral artery

The femoral artery is located level with your pubic bone, just beneath the crease in your groin between your thigh and lower abdomen.

How to do it

Compress the femoral artery with your fingers – fairly heavy pressure will be required. When you feel the flow has ceased, hold for 30 seconds. The blood will then back up and increase the pressure in the iliac arteries, which forces more blood into the pelvic arteries. This floods the pelvic organs with more blood. When the hold is released, you should feel a sensation of warmth rushing down your legs as the blood supply returns to the lower extremities.

Contraindications
Do not perform this exercise if you are pregnant, have high blood pressure, have heart disease or circulatory problems (aneurisms, varicose veins, phlebitis, thrombosis), have a history of strokes or detached retinas.

Mustard and turmeric poultice

A mustard poultice can be very effective in cases where over-the-counter heat patches help to soothe pain in conditions such as endometriosis. Turmeric is a potent anti-inflammatory – it helps to relieve pain and promotes healing. Caution: Mustard can 'burn' skin if it is in direct contact with it. To avoid this, wrap the poultice in a couple of layers of muslin or a face cloth before applying.

REFERENCES AND FURTHER READING

Beal, M. W. (1999) 'Acupuncture and acupressure: Applications to women's reproductive health care.' *Journal of Nurse-Midwifery 44*, 217–230.

Chen, Y. F., Zhang, C. Y., Zhang, X. Y. *et al.* (2008) 'Effects of acupuncture combined with medicine on expression of matrix metalloproteinase-2 in the rat of endometriosis.' *Zhongguo Zhen Jiu 28*, 675–680.

Ernst, E. (1996) 'Hypoglycaemic plant medicines.' *Perfusion 9*, 416–418.

Green, I., Cohen, S. L., Finkenzeller, D. and Christo, P. J. (2010) 'Interventional therapies for controlling pelvic pain: What is the evidence?' *Current Pain Headache Report 14*, 22–32.

Guo, A. and Meng, Q. (2008) 'Acupuncture combined with spinal tuina for treatment of primary dysmenorrhea in 30 cases.' *Journal of Traditional Chinese Medicine 28*, 7–9.

Guo, Z., Jia, X., Liu, J. P., Liao, J. and Yang, Y. (2012) 'Herbal medicines for advanced colorectal cancer.' *Cochrane Database of Systematic Reviews*.

Hu, G. Z. and Li, X. Y. (1995) '48 endometriosis patients treated by the principle of eliminating stagnation and activating blood circulation.' *Shanghai Journal of Traditional Chinese Medicine 2*, 38–40.

Iorno, V., Burani, R., Bianchini, B., Minelli, E., Martinelli, F. and Ciatto, S. (2008) 'Acupuncture treatment of dysmenorrhea resistant to conventional medical treatment.' *Evidence-Based Complementary and Alternative Medicine 5*, 227–230.

Jian, L., Xiangyun, L. and Xiaomei, X. (1998) 'Clinical observation on patients with endometriosis treated by tonifying kidney and removing blood stasis.' *Chinese Journal of Integrated Traditional and Western Medicine 4*, 3, 166–169.

Jingxi, Y. and Guodong, P. (1993) 'Review of pharmacology studies and applications of Xuefu Zhuyu Tang.' *Journal of the Shandong College of Traditional Chinese Medicine 17*, 6, 423–425.

Li, C. H., Wang, Y. Z. and Guo, X. Y. (2008) 'Acupuncture at Siguan points for treatment of primary dysmenorrhea.' *Zhongguo Zhen Jiu 28*, 187–190.

Lin, L. L., Liu, C. Z. and Huang, B. Y. (2008) 'Clinical observation on treatment of primary dysmenorrhea with acupuncture and massage.' *Zhongguo Zhong Xi Yi Jie He Za Zhi 28*, 418–420.

Missmer, S. A. (2010) 'A prospective study of dietary fat consumption and endometriosis risk.' *Human Reproduction*, March.

Shao, G. Q. (1980) 'Clinical and experimental research on 156 cases of endometriosis treated by therapy of promoting blood circulation and removing stasis.' *Shanghai Journal of Traditional Chinese Medicine 3*, 4–6.

Song, Y. H., Yu, J. and Yu, C. Q. (2005) 'Clinical observation of Yu's neiyi recipe: Combined Chinese herbs enema and external application in treating 36 patients with endometriosis.' *Zhongguo Zhong Xi Yi Jie He Za Zhi 25*, 748–749.

Temple, J. (2007) *The Genius of China: 3,000 Years of Science, Discovery, and Invention.* London: Prion Books Ltd.

Wang, D. G., Wang, Z. Q. and Zhang, Z. F. (1991) 'Treatment of endometriosis with removing blood-stasis and purgation method.' *Chinese Journal of Integrated Traditional and Western Medicine 11*, 9, 524–526.

Zhuang, B. and Xia, G. C. (1990) 'Correlation between treatment of syndrome differentiation and basic body temperature in 21 cases of endometriosis.' *Shanxi Journal of Traditional Chinese Medicine 11*, 12, 537.

Chapter 6

FIBROIDS

FIBROIDS IN BIOMEDICINE

It is estimated that over two-thirds of women of reproductive age will have fibroids, although many will never know as their fibroids are small enough not to cause symptoms (asymptomatic). Fibroids frequently go unnoticed until they grow rapidly during a perimenopausal phase around age 40, and most decline substantially after menopause (as the uterus shrinks, so do the fibroids). If a woman takes oestrogen after menopause, the fibroids may remain as they are or grow even larger.

Small fibroids usually have no symptoms, but larger masses can cause excessive menstrual bleeding, and very large fibroids can contribute to miscarriage, abdominal pain and profuse bleeding causing anaemia.

The exact cause of fibroids is unknown, but many doctors and researchers believe that fibroids grow in response to a number of primary and secondary factors that interact with a woman's unique genetic make-up, causing an imbalance within the body. Oestrogen levels are more than likely the overall primary factor. There are two key factors that support this theory:

- The large increases in local oestrogen concentration within a fibroid itself, and concentrations of oestrogen receptors in fibroid tissue are higher than in the surrounding tissue.

- The fact that fibroids shrink at menopause. At menopause a woman's circulating oestrogen levels decrease dramatically, but women who take supplemental oestrogen after menopause may still have issues with fibroids.

COMPLICATIONS

The most likely issue with uterine fibroids is bleeding, which can manifest as spotting or breakthrough bleeding of heavy periods.

Fibroids, if large enough, can press on the bladder in front of the uterus or on the rectum behind the uterus, causing either frequent urination or constipation.

Fibroids may interfere with the ability to become pregnant if they bulge into the interior of the uterus, and large uterine fibroids may be responsible for early-stage miscarriages.

FIBROIDS IN CHINESE MEDICINE

The first depiction of uterine fibroids in the Chinese literature was in the *Ling Shu*, which defined shijia, a stony tumour (shi = stone, jia = mass). From this text arose the general concept of abdominal masses as zhengjia, which denotes two types of masses: Zheng refers to one in fixed position that is painful, and Jia is a mass that can be moved, and only hurts when pressure is applied.

In the *Jingui Yaolue* (*Essential Prescriptions from the Golden Cabinet*, 1340), the situation was described whereby menstrual bleeding would cease for three months, followed by incessant bleeding, indicating that a mass had formed. This scenario is consistent with the concept that the womb is blocked and obstructed (hence the lack of bleeding), but then it develops a mass, which causes the incessant bleeding.

In most cases fibroids are characterised by an accumulation of fluid (Dampness or Phlegm) either locally or systemically. Foods that have a diuretic (fluid draining) action are important in reducing the size of fibroids.

The addition of spices that move Qi in the smaller vessels is also important as normal Qi flow will help keep fluids moving and prevent stagnation occurring in the first place.

DIETARY CONSIDERATIONS

The idea is to exclude foods from your diet that are likely to encourage excess oestrogen production. The most important dietary recommendations are to eat a high fibre diet rich in phytoestrogens while avoiding saturated fat, sugar and caffeine.

Phytoestrogens (plant estrogens) are able to bind to the same cell receptors as the oestrogen your body produces. Phytoestrogens occupy the oestrogen receptor sites in your cells, preventing a need for production of more oestrogen. As fibroids and the tissue surrounding them are likely to have the most receptor sites, they are the first to be affected. Phytoestrogens bind to the receptors in the fibroid preventing any of the oestrogen gaining access. This, combined with the drop in oestrogen production, starves the fibroid, which will begin to shrink.

Phytonutrients found in cruciferous vegetables such as cabbage, turnips or Brussels sprouts are very effective at breaking down surplus oestrogens. These phytonutrients (indole-3-carbinol (I3C), diindoylmethane (DIM) and sulfurophane) are often the active ingredients in anti-fibroid nutritional formulas sold on the internet.

The ideal anti-fibroid diet is mostly vegetarian with small amounts of high-quality meat or fish.

VITAMIN AND MINERAL SUPPLEMENTS

Vitamin D: In animal studies vitamin D caused existing fibroids to shrink as well as preventing new fibroids growing. In a study performed by the Meharry Medical College in Nashville, Tennessee, vitamin D supplementation inhibited the growth of fibroid cells by 47 per cent (Sharan *et al.* 2010).

Iron: Uterine fibroids can cause heavy menstrual bleeding and resultant anaemia. If you find over-the-counter iron supplements cause constipation, try black strap molasses. Add it to warm water or put it on your porridge in the morning.

Magnesium citrate: Uterine fibroids can become calcified (stone-like). Magnesium supplements dissolve the calcium layer around the fibroids and fully eliminate the calcified layer, thus preventing the calcification of uterine fibroid tumours.

THERAPEUTIC RECIPES

For a complete listing of the energetic qualities and uses in Chinese medicine of most common foods, see Appendix A.

Breakfast

Porridge made with water and sprinkled with cinnamon. Porridge is warming in nature; it improves digestive function and Blood circulation. Cinnamon improves Blood circulation in the smaller vessels such as those in the fingers, toes or around the reproductive organs. Adding black strap molasses will help prevent anaemia due to excessive blood loss, as it is high in iron.

Walnuts and/or cashews in natural yoghurt. Although yoghurt is considered cold in nature, both walnuts and cashews are warming. It is important to choose yoghurt with no added sugar and live bacteria.

Lunch

Salad: Many salad vegetables are cold in nature (this can slow down digestive function and impair the movement of Qi and Blood), but the addition of onions, garlic, ginger, chilli or peppers can mediate the cooling action of the vegetables.

Try some of the following combinations:

Carrot, apple and ginger

Carrot and radish

Duck, watercress and orange

Guacamole

Mixed beans with chilli

Prawns with bean sprouts

Dinner

MUNG BEAN AND CABBAGE SOUP

Ingredients

- 3 tbsp olive oil
- 1 small onion, finely chopped
- 3 cloves garlic, grated or finely chopped
- 150 g (5 oz) mung beans
- 2 tsp turmeric

- 2 tsp ground cumin
- 3 tsp coriander seeds, toasted and ground
- 100 g (3½ oz) cabbage, shredded
- sea salt and black pepper

Method

1. In a large pan, heat the olive oil and add the onion. Cook until the onions are soft.

2. Add the garlic and cook for another minute.

3. Add the mung beans and spices.

4. Add enough water to cover the mung beans and cook until tender.

5. Add the cabbage and cook for a further 5 minutes.

6. Season to taste. Serve.

Therapeutic qualities

Mung beans: Drain Dampness (excess fluid).

Cabbage: Drains Dampness by promoting urination. The sweet taste nourishes the Spleen, the origin of Blood; this is important in cases where there is anaemia from heavy bleeding.

Garlic, onion, black pepper, coriander and cumin: Are all aromatic in nature; they transform Dampness and move Qi.

Turmeric: Moves Qi while draining Dampness (inflammation).

PEARL BARLEY AND CHICKPEA SOUP

Ingredients

- 1 tsp olive oil
- 1 small onion, diced
- 1 carrot, diced
- 1 stalk celery, diced
- 1 parsnip, diced
- 400 g (14 oz) tin chopped tomatoes

- 1.8 litres (8 cups) vegetable or chicken stock
- 400 g (14 oz) tin chickpeas (garbanzo beans), drained and rinsed
- 40 g (2 oz) pearl barley
- 30 g (1½ oz) kale, shredded
- sea salt and black pepper

Method

1. In a pan heat the oil and sauté the onion, carrot, celery and parsnip until soft.

2. Add the tin of chopped tomatoes, the stock, chickpeas and barley.

3. Bring to the boil, reduce to a simmer and cook for about 25 minutes.

4. Add the kale and cook for another 10 minutes.

5. Season and serve.

Therapeutic qualities

Chickpeas: Stimulate diuresis.

Celery: Clears Heat and detoxifies.

Carrots: Clear Heat and nourish Blood (high vitamin A content).

Kale: Tonifies Qi.

Tomatoes: Clear Heat and nourish Body Fluids.

Parsnips: Blood tonic as well as drying Dampness.

CHICKPEA CURRY

Ingredients

- 1 tbsp olive oil
- 1 onion, chopped
- 1 garlic clove, grated or finely chopped
- ¼ tsp sea salt
- ½ tsp ground cumin
- ¼ tsp ground coriander
- ¼ tsp ground turmeric
- ¼ tsp red chilli powder

- 1 fresh tomato, chopped
- 400 g (14 oz) tin chickpeas (garbanzo beans), drained and rinsed
- 5 cm (2 inches) fresh root ginger, grated or finely chopped
- 1 tsp five spice powder (see below)

FIVE SPICE POWDER

- 1 tsp ground cinnamon
- 1 tsp ground cloves
- 1 tsp Szechuan peppercorns, toasted and ground

- 1 tsp fennel seeds, toasted and ground
- 1 tsp ground star anise

Method

1. Begin by mixing together the ingredients for the five spice powder. It will make more than you need for this recipe, but will store in an airtight jar for months.

2. Heat the oil in a wok or lidded frying pan. Fry the onion and garlic until caramelised.

3. Add the salt, cumin, coriander, turmeric and red chilli powder. Mix for a minute and add the tomato. Cook until the sauce begins to thicken.

4. Add 4 tbsp water and stir. Then add the chickpeas and mix. Mash a few of the chickpeas while cooking. Cover and simmer for 5 minutes.

5. Add the ginger and five spice powder and cook for another minute. Serve.

Therapeutic qualities

Chickpeas: Drain Dampness by stimulating diuresis.

Onion, garlic, chilli and ginger: All drain Dampness due to their aromatic nature. They reinforce the Damp-draining action of the chickpeas.

Tomato: Builds Body Fluids. It is important that as stagnant waste fluids are cleared from the body that 'clean' pure fluids are replenished.

Turmeric: Moves Qi while draining Dampness (inflammation). Curcumin, the active ingredient in turmeric, is a potent anti-inflammatory.

Cumin and coriander: Regulate Qi flow. Movement of Qi is important, as lack of free movement is what allows the pooling of Body Fluids (resulting in Dampness/Phlegm) in the first place.

Five spice: Cinnamon moves Qi and Blood in the smaller vessels, cloves break Blood stasis, Szechuan peppercorns tonify Qi, fennel seeds envoy to the lower Jiao and star anise tonifies Qi.

 ## ROAST VEGETABLES WITH FIVE SPICE

Ingredients

- 1 butternut squash (or pumpkin), cut into bite-size cubes
- 2 red peppers (bell peppers), seeded and diced
- 1 sweet potato, peeled and diced
- 3 potatoes, diced (skins on or off, it's up to you)
- 1 red onion, quartered
- olive oil
- 2 tsp five spice powder (see above)
- 2 tbsp balsamic vinegar
- sea salt

Method

1. Preheat the oven to 200°C/Gas Mark 6/400°F.

2. In a large bowl, combine the squash, red pepper, sweet potato, potatoes and red onion.

3. On a baking tray add the olive oil, vinegar and five spice powder, and toss the vegetables in the mix until coated. Spread the vegetables out evenly on the tray. Add the balsamic vinegar and a sprinkle of sea salt.

4. Roast until the vegetables are cooked through and slightly browned. Serve.

Therapeutic qualities

Squash/pumpkin: Clears Heat and drains Dampness by promoting diuresis.

Onion and peppers: Assist the squash in draining Dampness.

Sweet potato: Their sweet nature harmonises the digestive system (in excess they can damage it).

Potato: Their sweet nature harmonises the digestive system (in excess they can damage it).

Balsamic vinegar: Its sweet/astringent nature assists the potatoes in harmonising the digestive system.

Five spice mix: Cinnamon moves Qi and Blood in the smaller vessels, cloves break Blood stasis, Szechuan peppercorns tonify Qi, fennel seeds envoy to the lower Jiao and star anise tonifies Qi. The warm spicy nature of the five spice powder moderates the cooling nature of the squash and the Damp-forming tendencies of the potatoes.

 ## PRAWN CURRY

Ingredients

- 1 tbsp vegetable oil
- ½ onion, finely sliced
- 2 cm (⅘ inch) fresh root ginger, grated or finely chopped
- 1 clove garlic, grated or finely chopped
- 1 tomato, diced
- 1 tsp five spice powder (see above)
- 1 tsp cayenne pepper
- sea salt
- 100 ml (3½ fl oz) coconut milk
- 100 ml (3½ fl oz) water
- 1 chilli, chopped
- 6 king prawns (or 150 g (5 oz) trout fillets)

Method

1. Heat the oil in a pan and add the onion, ginger and garlic. Fry until soft and fragrant.
2. Add the tomato, five spice powder, cayenne pepper and salt, and fry until the spices are aromatic.
3. Pour in the coconut milk, water and chopped chilli. When the mixture comes to a good boil, add the king prawns (or trout fillets) and cook until they are cooked through. Serve straight away.

Therapeutic qualities

Prawns: Tonify Kidney Qi. Trout will have the same Qi tonifying effect.

Cayenne pepper: Tonifies Qi and reinforces the tonifying action of the prawns.

Ginger, garlic, onion and chilli: All dispel Dampness due to their aromatic nature. Ginger and chilli also move Blood and prevent stasis.

Coconut milk: Nourishes Blood while moving Qi.

Tomato: Clears Heat and builds Body Fluids.

Five spice powder: Cinnamon moves Qi and Blood in the smaller vessels, cloves break Blood stasis, Szechuan peppercorns tonify Qi, fennel seeds envoy to the lower Jiao and star anise tonifies Qi.

 ## CHICKEN AND VEGETABLE STEW

Ingredients

- 1 tbsp olive oil
- 1 onion, finely chopped
- 1 leek, finely sliced
- 2 cloves garlic, grated or finely chopped
- 2 carrots, diced
- 1 parsnip, peeled and chopped
- 2 sticks celery, diced
- 4 chicken thighs, skin removed
- 100 g (3½ oz) pearl barley
- 2 bay leaves
- 300 ml (10 fl oz) chicken stock

Method

1. Heat the oil in a large casserole dish or saucepan and fry the onion and leek for 5 minutes before adding the garlic for a further minute.

2. Add all the other ingredients, giving everything a good stir. Bring to a simmer, put the lid on and allow to cook slowly for 45 minutes. Serve.

Therapeutic qualities

Pearl barley: Drains Dampness.

Bay leaves: Harmonise the Stomach and Intestines, dispel Dampness.

Parsnip, leek, onion and celery: Dispel Dampness.

Garlic: Moves Blood and aids in draining Dampness due to its aromatic nature.

All the foods reinforce the pearl barley's Damp-draining action.

Chicken: Tonifies Qi. Qi is needed to provide the motive force to propel Dampness from the body.

Carrots: Build and move Blood. The combination of carrot and garlic in this recipe will gently move Blood and prevent Blood stasis.

 QUINOA AND BLACK BEANS

Ingredients

- 1 tsp vegetable oil
- 1 onion, finely chopped
- 3 cloves garlic, grated or finely chopped
- 100 g (3½ oz) quinoa
- 2 tsp ground cumin
- 1 tsp cayenne pepper
- 300 ml (10 fl oz) vegetable or chicken stock
- 400 g (14 oz) tin black beans, rinsed and drained

Method

1. Heat the oil in a pan over a medium heat, then cook the onion and garlic until softened but not brown.

2. Add the quinoa and spices to the pan and stir for a minute.

3. Add the stock, bring the mixture to a boil, cover, reduce the heat and simmer until the quinoa is tender and the stock is absorbed.

4. Add the black beans and warm through. Serve.

Therapeutic qualities

Quinoa: Kidney Qi tonic; it will increase Qi circulation in the whole body.

Black beans: Kidney Qi tonic and diuretic.

Cumin: Harmonises the Stomach and Intestines. Cumin combined with garlic and onion reinforces the diuretic action of the black beans.

Cayenne pepper: Qi tonic. It supports the Qi tonifying action of quinoa and black beans.

Onions and garlic: Their aromatic nature means that they dispel Dampness. Garlic is also an excellent herb to keep Blood moving, preventing stagnation.

ACUPRESSURE

How to apply pressure to the points

To press points, use something blunt. You can use finger pressure, but if you have to apply sustained pressure, you may find it uncomfortable. A chopstick (like the ones you get with a takeaway meal) is ideal for this purpose.

Ideally have someone do the treatment for you; that way you are not creating muscular tension while you try and reach points. You can also focus more on what sensations (or lack of them) result from pressing the point.

Don't press too hard; use enough pressure that you (or your partner) can feel something happening.

When you get to the point where something is happening, keep the pressure constant and hold for 30 seconds.

If you are not feeling any effects from pressing a point, you may not be pressing on the exact right spot. Try different spots around the location you first tried.

The points

There are any number of points that can be used, and in most cases points used in an acupuncture treatment are selected based on signs and symptoms presenting at that time. The points listed below are all useful in the treatment of fibroids, but for a more individualised treatment plan, talk to a licensed acupuncture practitioner.

LUNG 1 (ZHONG FU) CENTRAL TREASURY

Actions – Transforms Phlegm and regulates the water passages.

Location – At the level of the first intercostal space (the space between your ribs), six finger breadths from your breastbone.

Location note – The first space that you come to above your ribcage is the top of the first rib.

SAN JIAO 10 (TIAN JING) CELESTIAL WELL

Actions – Transforms Phlegm and dissipates nodules.

Location – When the elbow is flexed the point is in the depression about one finger breadth superior to the olecranon (the point of your elbow).

STOMACH 28 (SHUI DAO) WATERWAY

Actions – Regulates the lower Jiao and dispels stagnation; benefits the Bladder and the uterus.

Location – Three finger breadths below the umbilicus, two finger breadths lateral to the midline.

STOMACH 32 (FU TU) CROUCHING RABBIT

Actions – *Sagelike Prescriptions from the Taiping Era* recommends Stomach 32 for treating diseases of the eight regions in women. These are the external genitals, the internal genitals, the breast, disorders of pregnancy, post-partum disorders, uterine bleeding, leucorrhoea menstruation and abdominal masses.

Location – Put your hand on the outside edge of your hip and you will feel a curve in the bone (the anterior superior iliac spine). Imagine a line joining this bone and the outside edge of your kneecap. The point is eight finger breadths along this line when measured from the top of the kneecap up.

STOMACH 40 (FENG LONG) ABUNDANT BULGE

Actions – Transforms Phlegm.

Location – Approximately half-way between the lower edge of your kneecap and the ankle crease two finger breadths from the outside edge of your shin bone. In most people it lives up to its name and you can feel the bulge.

SPLEEN 15 (DA HENG) GREAT HORIZONTAL

Actions – Moves Qi and regulates the Intestines.

Location – On the abdomen in the depression at the lateral border of the rectus abdominis muscle level with the umbilicus.

Location note – The point is one hand's breadth from your belly button on the same level.

REFERENCES AND FURTHER READING

Catherino, W. H., Malik, M., Britten, J., Gilden, M., Segars, J. and McCarthy-Keith, D. (2010) 'Leiomyoma fibrosis inhibited by liarozole, a retinoic acid metabolic blocking agent.' *Fertility and Sterility 94*, 4, S32–S33.

Du, W. H. (1993) 'Retentive enema and oral taking of Guizhi Fuling Wan for treatment of 40 cases of uterine fibroids.' *Shandong Journal of Traditional Chinese Medicine 12*, 2, 28–29.

Hsu, H. Y. (1984) 'Chinese herb therapy for uterine myomas.' *Bulletin of the Oriental Healing Arts Institute 9*, 6, 294–298.

Huali, P. (1989) 'Treatment of hysteromyoma with Gui Ling Xiaoliu Wan: A report of 30 cases.' *Beijing Journal of Traditional Chinese Medicine 6*, 30–31.

Jiang, P., Zhao, Y., Ruan, Y. L. and Han, Y. (2003) 'Clinical observation of 70 cases of hysteromyoma treated with integrated traditional Chinese and Western medicine.' *Modern Journal of Integrated Traditional Chinese and Western Medicine 12*, 7, 707–708.

Kang, Y. P. and Zheng, S. G. (2005) '46 cases of hysteromyoma at early stage treated with integrated traditional Chinese and Western medicine.' *Shaanxi Journal of Traditional Chinese Medicine 26*, 5, 402–403.

Liu, W. M., Ng, H. T., Wu, Y. C., Yen, Y. K. and Yuan, C. C. (2001) 'Laparoscopic bipolar coagulation of uterine vessels: A new method for treating symptomatic fibroids.' *Fertility and Sterility 75*, 2, 417–422.

Lu, J. X. (2007) 'Comparison of Huoxue Sanjie Decoction with mifepristone in the treatment of uterine fibroids.' *Shandong Journal of Medicine and Pharmacology 47*, 19, 109–110.

Lu, Y. and Deng, Z. H. (2005) 'Clinical observation on the treatment of hysteromyoma with Qi-stagnancy and blood-stasis syndrome with Huazheng Decoction.' *Journal of Anhui Traditional Chinese Medical College 24*, 6, 16–17.

Medikare, V., Kandukuri, L. R., Ananthapur, V., Deenadayal, M. and Nallari, P. (2011) 'The genetic bases of uterine fibroids: A review.' *Journal of Reproduction & Infertility 12*, 3, 181–191.

Okolo, S. (2008) 'Incidence, aetiology and epidemiology of uterine fibroids.' *Clinical Obstetrics & Gynaecology 22*, 4, 571–587.

Sharan, C., Halder, S. K., Thota, C., Jaleel, T., Nair, S. and Al-Hendy, A. (2010) *Vitamin D Inhibits Proliferation of Human Uterine Leiomyoma Cells Via Catechol-Omethyltransferase.* Nashville, TN: Meharry Medical College.

Wang, H. (2010) *Sagelike Prescriptions from the Taiping Era (Taiping Shenghui Fang).* Beijing, China: Institute for the History of Natural Science, China Academy of Sciences.

Zhuen, Z. (2000) 'Clinical observation of 28 cases of hysteromyoma healed by integrated traditional and Western medicine.' *Chinese Journal of Integrated Traditional and Western Medicine 13*, 3, 180–181.

Chapter 7

INFERTILITY

INFERTILITY IN CHINESE MEDICINE

Chinese medicine has a long history in treating infertility. Chapter 1 of the *Huangdi Neijing* (*The Yellow Emperor's Classic of Internal Medicine*) describes the various stages of a woman's life. It almost exactly mirrors the biomedical model in stating that at age 28 fertility reaches its apex and begins its shift toward menopause by the age of 49.

There are a number of conditions that can contribute to infertility that are examined below, and the menstrual cycle itself is always a good starting point.

THE MENSTRUAL CYCLE IN BIOMEDICINE

A menstrual cycle can be divided into four main phases:

- Menstrual, day 1 to 5

- Follicular, day 1 to 13

- Ovulation, day 14

- Luteal, day 15 to 28

The days corresponding to the stages of the cycle are approximate and based on a 28-day cycle. If your cycle is longer or shorter, don't worry – consistency is the main thing.

Menstrual phase, day 1 to 5

The menstrual phase begins on the first day of a period and lasts until the fifth day of the menstrual cycle. Regardless of whether a period lasts until day 5, this is still regarded as the menstrual phase.

During this phase the uterus sheds its inner lining of soft tissue and blood vessels, resulting in blood loss of somewhere between 10 and 80 ml (0.3 and 3 fl oz).

Oestrogen and progesterone levels are at their lowest during this time of the menstrual cycle.

Follicular phase, day 1 to 13

This phase also begins on the first day of a period and lasts about 10 to 14 days, or until ovulation occurs.

The follicle-stimulating hormone (FSH) is secreted by the anterior pituitary gland. The rise in FSH levels causes the growth of a number of follicles (a sac-like structure that contains an egg(s)) that then compete with each other for dominance. These follicles are found along the outside layer of the ovaries and eggs (oocytes) that have been in a half-developed dormant state waiting to develop to maturity from within a follicle. In a typical menstrual cycle only one follicle reaches maturity.

- It takes approximately 13 days for the egg cell to reach maturity.

- While the egg cell matures, a surge of oestrogen produced by the ovaries stimulates the uterus to develop a lining of blood vessels and soft tissue (endometrium).

- Once the levels of oestrogen are at their peak, the pituitary gland slows the secretion of FSH, and instead begins to secrete the luteinising hormone (LH). As a result of the increase in LH, the mature follicle ruptures and releases the egg (ovum).

Ovulation phase, day 14

The released egg cell is swept into the fallopian tube by the cilia of the fimbriae. (Fimbriae are finger-like projections located at the end of the fallopian tube close to the ovaries, and cilia are hair-like projections on each fimbria.)

For the remainder of the cycle, the remnants of the ovarian follicle form a corpus luteum. LH stimulates the corpus luteum to produce progesterone that is required to support the early stages of pregnancy, if fertilisation occurs.

Luteal phase, day 15 to 28
This phase begins on the 15th day and lasts until the end of the cycle.

- The egg cell released during the ovulation phase stays in the fallopian tube for 24 hours.

- If a sperm cell does not impregnate the egg cell within that time, the egg cell disintegrates.

- If conception and implantation do not occur, the pituitary gland will reduce LH and FSH production. Without the presence of LH, the corpus luteum deteriorates and the oestrogen and progesterone levels subsequently decrease. The drop in oestrogen and progesterone levels triggers the shedding of the endometrium, causing menstruation to begin, and the cycle starts over again.

THE MENSTRUAL CYCLE IN CHINESE MEDICINE

In Chinese medicine a menstrual cycle is broken down into a Yin and Yang cycle.

Yin cycle
Follicular phase

- Day 1: Levels of oestrogen and progesterone fall and the endometrium starts to shed. Chong Mai (Sea of Blood) starts to empty of Blood (see the 'Channel theory' section in Chapter 4).

- Day 3: New endometrium is being established (while still shedding the old). This is governed by the Chong and Ren Mai (Sea of Blood and Directing Vessel).

- Day 5: Rebuilding of the endometrium is complete. Rising oestrogen levels promote more endometrial growth that reflects the refilling of the Chong Mai (Sea of Blood).

Follicles
From day 1 follicles in the ovary start to grow.

Yin or Blood deficiency will cause the follicles to take longer to mature, will delay ovulation and menstrual cycles will be longer. In biomedicine this can equate to poor oestrogen production, reduced sensitivity to FSH or poor FSH production by the pituitary gland.

Mid-cycle phase
Yin is at its peak Chong Mai (Sea of Blood) (and the uterus) are full of Blood.

Around day 14 oestrogen levels peak for 48 hours and a surge of LH from the pituitary gland triggers ovulation. Progesterone starts to be produced from the corpus luteum. Both these events signal the start of the Yang part of the cycle.

Yang cycle
Luteal phase
The corpus luteum produces progesterone under the influence of LH.

The corpus luteum peaks in size to 1.5 cm (0.6 inches) one week after ovulation (approximately day 21) under the initial surge of LH. If LH levels drop, the corpus luteum will degenerate, progesterone levels will drop and by day 28 the endometrium breaks down and produces a period.

The high progesterone levels will cause the basal body temperature (BBT) to rise; it should remain high for 14 days after ovulation.

INFERTILITY: THE BASIC FACTS
The NHS states that approximately 84 per cent of couples will conceive naturally within one year if they have regular unprotected sex.

For every 100 couples trying to conceive naturally:

- 84 will conceive within one year

- 92 will conceive within two years

- 93 will conceive within three years.

For couples who have been trying to conceive for more than three years without success, the likelihood of pregnancy occurring within the next year is 25 per cent or less.

It is generally recommended that if you have failed to conceive after one year of unprotected sex, seek advice. If you are over 35, seek advice after six months.

COMMON CAUSES OF INFERTILITY

Female issues are responsible in up to 45 per cent of cases. These can include:

- Endometriosis

- Endocrine (hormonal) issues

- Poor ovarian reserve

- Polycystic ovarian syndrome (PCOS)

- Fallopian tube blockages.

Male issues are responsible in up to 30 per cent of cases. These can include:

- Obstruction of the vas deferens or epididymis, the tubes that carry sperm. Blockages can be caused by infection, such as chlamydia, gonorrhoea or traumatic injury.

- Varicoceles (enlarged veins in the scrotum) can affect sperm production by disrupting normal testicular function.

- Sperm quality: No sperm present (azoospermia), low sperm count (oligozoospermia), poor sperm motility (asthenospermia) or abnormally shaped sperm (morphology).

- Anti-sperm antibodies: Some men have an immune reaction to semen, which causes them to produce anti-sperm antibodies that damage their sperm. This is most common after a vasectomy reversal.

Unexplained sub-fertility is diagnosed in about 40 per cent of cases. This is a diagnosis of exclusion and is usually made after investigations show nothing is definitively wrong with either partner. This is the diagnosis that causes the greatest stress as it is so vague; at least with the other diagnoses there is a known pathogen or physical issue, which is not so in this case.

BASAL BODY TEMPERATURE CHARTS

Though many Western practitioners find basal body temperature (BBT) charts to be unnecessary in their practices, these readings can provide useful insights about your cycle for Chinese medicine practitioners specialising in fertility.

BBT chart fluctuations reflect changes in hormone levels at different stages of the menstrual cycle.

During pre-ovulation (follicular phase), temperatures should remain fairly stable (most people average 36 degrees). Typically, there is a dip in BBT when LH surges just before ovulation, and a spike in temperature shortly after ovulation.

These dips and peaks are visible on BBT charts, as long as you use an accurate thermometer. To take an accurate BBT reading:

- You need at least 3–4 hours of unbroken sleep (insomnia causes higher BBT).

- Use a digital thermometer (you can buy a BBT thermometer).

- Take your temperature at the same time each morning (even at the weekends).

- BBT rises roughly 0.1°C each hour after rising (to calculate back if necessary).

- Start charting on day 1 of your period.

- Chart for at least three whole cycles to establish the BBT pattern through a cycle.

- BBT level at ovulation should show a thermal shift upwards of at least 0.4°C.

- BBT temperature should remain elevated (varying no more than 0.1°C) for at least 12–14 days of the luteal period.

Factors that can push up BBT artificially

- Insomnia: Look for the temperature your body reaches when cooled at complete rest (BBT). To get to this point will take at least 3 hours of unbroken sleep.

- Drinking alcohol: Alcohol can disrupt hormonal processes and lead to artificial spikes in BBT.

- Fever: Your BBT will be artificially high if you have a fever.

THE ORAL CONTRACEPTIVE PILL AND FERTILITY

The oral contraceptive pill works by suppressing the pituitary gland's cyclic excretion of hormones that stimulates the release of eggs from your ovaries. It does this by using combinations of synthetic oestrogen and progesterone, so your body is fooled into thinking it is pregnant and this prevents the release of an egg every month. The issue with this is that your own normal hormonal cycle is thrown out of balance. In many cases it will re-establish itself within a couple of cycles after you stop taking the pill. However, if you have previously suffered from either endometriosis or PCOS, regulating your cycle may prove a little more troublesome.

When looked at from a Chinese medicine viewpoint the oral contraceptive pill induces a condition of Qi stagnation – what should move in a predictable cycle (hormones) cannot move, and this suppression induces stagnation. In cases where there are underlying pathologies involving Blood stasis or Phlegm/Dampness, the Qi stagnation exacerbates the problem.

SELF-HELP FOR INFERTILITY

- Incorporate more fibre into your diet: A high fibre diet (30 g (1 oz) a day) can improve bowel function, allowing unmetabolised hormones to be cleared from the system.

- Do a liver detox: Your liver regulates hormonal function; if it is impaired, endocrine (hormone) imbalances can occur.

- Exercise: Physical activity can help move stagnant Liver Qi.

ACUPRESSURE

How to apply pressure to the points

To press points, use something blunt. You can use finger pressure, but if you have to apply sustained pressure, you may find it uncomfortable. A chopstick (like the ones you get with a takeaway meal) is ideal for this purpose.

Ideally have someone do the treatment for you; that way you are not creating muscular tension while you try and reach points. You can also focus more on what sensations (or lack of them) result from pressing the point.

Don't press too hard; use enough pressure that you (or your partner) can feel something happening.

When you get to the point where something is happening, keep the pressure constant and hold for 30 seconds.

If you are not feeling any effects from pressing a point, you may not be pressing on the exact right spot. Try different spots around the location you first tried.

The points

There are any number of points that can be used, and in most cases points used in an acupuncture treatment are selected based on signs and symptoms presenting at that time. The points listed below are all useful, but for a more individualised treatment plan, talk to a licensed acupuncture practitioner.

The following point combination is one I find effective in clinic to help balance out fluctuating hormone levels. The first two points used in combination are often referred to as the 'Four Gates' – they open up the various aspects (gates) of the body and mind, and allow proper integrated function within the self.

LARGE INTESTINE 4 (HE GU) PEACEFUL VALLEY

Actions – Moves Qi and Blood.

Location – On the dorsum of the hand between the first and second metacarpal bones, approximately in the middle of the second metacarpal bone on the radial side.

Location note – Between the thumb and first finger, just above the web.

Caution – This point can induce labour, so do not use if you are pregnant.

LIVER 3 (TAI CHONG) GREAT SURGE

Actions – Smooths the flow of Qi, nourishes Blood, regulates menstruation and regulates the lower abdominal and pelvic regions.

Location – On the dorsum of the foot in the depression distal to the junction of the first and second metatarsal bones.

Location note – Run your finger back from the web between your big and second toe. The point is at the junction of the bones that your finger runs into.

REN 4 (GUAN YUAN) ORIGIN PASS

Actions – Tonifies the Kidneys, benefits the uterus and assists conception.

Location – On the midline, three finger breadths below the umbilicus.

SPLEEN 6 (SAN YIN JIAO) THREE YIN INTERSECTION

Actions – Regulates menstruation, benefits the genitals, invigorates Blood, activates the Channel and alleviates pain.

Location – Three finger breadths directly above the tip of the medial malleolus posterior to the medial border of the tibia.

Location note – The point is three finger breadths above the round bone on the inside of your ankle, midway between the edge of the shin bone and Achilles tendon.

Caution – This point can induce labour, so do not use if you are pregnant.

DIMINISHED OVARIAN RESERVE

An ovarian reserve is a measure of the remaining number of eggs in a woman's ovaries. During your reproductive years the number of viable (good quality) eggs falls every month, and after the age of 35 it falls at an accelerated rate. While there is a strong correlation between age and ovarian reserve, the one does not necessarily follow the other – many older women have a strong ovarian reserve, while some younger women do not. Regardless of age it is an increase in FSH that contributes to diminished ovarian reserve. FSH is produced by the pituitary gland. This hormone is responsible for the growth of the egg within the ovaries each month. In younger women who usually have a large reserve of good quality eggs, small amounts of FSH are sufficient to stimulate the eggs to grow. As women age and egg quality and quantity decline, the pituitary needs to produce more and more FSH in order to stimulate egg growth. Simply put, the fewer eggs a woman has remaining in her reserve, the more FSH is needed to accomplish stimulation and growth, so in women whose ovarian reserve has declined, FSH levels climb higher and higher.

ELEVATED FOLLICLE-STIMULATING HORMONE AND HOW IT AFFECTS FERTILITY

FSH is typically measured in the early follicular phase of the menstrual cycle, typically day 3 to 5, counted from the last menstruation. At this time, the levels of estradiol and progesterone are at the lowest point of the menstrual cycle. FSH levels in this time are often called basal FSH levels, to distinguish them from the increased levels when approaching ovulation.

Elevated FSH can be defined as an FSH value of over 10 mg/dl (approx. 2 tsp) on day 3 of a woman's menstrual cycle.

Each laboratory establishes its own reference ranges, which is reflected in the differences from lab to lab. The specific reference ranges that appear on your laboratory report are determined and provided by the laboratory that performed your test.

In general, the following numbers and predictions occur:

Less than 10: This would be considered normal, and your response to stimulation should be good.

10–12: You have a slightly reduced ovarian reserve, which means that you will likely experience a reduced response to stimulation and possibly some reduction in egg and embryo quality.

12–16: There is a large reduction in eggs (and resulting embryo quality). Your response to stimulation may be quite poor.

Over 17: A very poor response or no response to stimulation.

Over 30: You are approaching or have begun menopause.

HIGH FOLLICLE-STIMULATING HORMONE LEVELS AND CHINESE MEDICINE

High FSH levels tend to result in diminished Blood flow to the ovaries and reproductive organs, leading to symptoms such as hot flushes, night sweats, vaginal dryness and menstrual irregularity. These symptoms all correlate with a Yin deficiency pattern. The broth recipe below is an excellent way to treat this.

BONE MARROW BROTH

Ingredients

- 1 kg (4 lbs) chicken or beef bones
- 1 pig's foot (optional)
- 1 large onion, roughly chopped
- 2 carrots, peeled and roughly chopped
- Enough water to cover the bones
- 3 stalks celery, roughly chopped
- 2 tbsp apple cider vinegar
- 40 g (2 oz) goji berries

Method

1. Preheat the oven to 200°C/Gas Mark 6/400°F.

2. Place the bones, pig's foot (if using), onion and carrot on a roasting pan and roast for 20 minutes. Toss the contents of the pan and roast for a further 20 minutes until deeply browned.

3. Scrape the bones and vegetables into a large stockpot and fill with enough water to cover. Add the celery, apple cider vinegar and the goji berries.

4. Cover the pot and bring to a gentle boil. Reduce heat to a low simmer and cook with the lid slightly ajar, skimming foam and

excess fat for at least 8, but up to, 24 hours (you can continue cooking it the following day).

5. Remove the pot from the heat and strain. The broth can be stored in the fridge for up to five days or in the freezer for up to six months.

Therapeutic qualities

Bones: Nourish Yin (the body's ability to cool and lubricate itself).

Pig's foot: Nourishes Yin.

Carrots and goji berries: Tonify Blood.

Onion: Provides aromatic warmth to balance out the cooling nature of the soup.

Vinegar: Helps leech out the minerals from the bones into the water.

SELF-HELP TREATMENTS

Ovarian massage

The ovaries lie approximately 10 cm (4 inches) down from the navel and 7 cm (2.7 inches) from the midline.

Massage the area in a circular motion; apply as much pressure as you can without causing pain. Pressure can be applied with your fingertips in a circular, kneading motion.

Fallopian tube massage

The fallopian tubes lie approximately 20 cm (8 inches) down from the navel and 5 cm (2 inches) out from the midline. (The uterus is on the midline.)

Massage this area in a clockwise outward direction using your fingertips. Make small clockwise circles with your fingertips as you massage outward for 10 to 15 cm (4 to 6 inches) on each side of the midline.

If you find areas of tension or tenderness, apply as much pressure as you can tolerate without causing pain. Focus more attention on massaging these tender spots.

If you are trying to get pregnant, this massage should only be practised between the end of a period and ovulation.

Femoral massage

This massage increases the blood flow to your pelvic organs. This increased blood flow may be useful in clearing any stagnations in the pelvic region (many acupuncture or herbal treatments will be trying to accomplish the same thing, albeit a bit more forcefully).

Locating your femoral artery

The femoral artery is located level with your pubic bone, just beneath the crease in your groin between your thigh and lower abdomen.

How to do it

Compress the femoral artery with your fingers – fairly heavy pressure will be required. When you feel the flow has ceased, hold for 30 seconds. The blood will then back up and increase the pressure in the iliac arteries, which forces more blood into the pelvic arteries. This floods the pelvic organs with more blood. When the hold is released, you should feel a sensation of warmth rushing down your legs as the blood supply returns to the lower extremities.

Contraindications

Do not perform this exercise if you are pregnant, have high blood pressure, have heart disease or circulatory problems (aneurisms, varicose veins, phlebitis, thrombosis), have a history of strokes or detached retinas.

THIN ENDOMETRIAL LINING

The uterus consists of three layers, and the innermost layer is known as the endometrium, which is the layer that is shed during a period. It is also the layer that thickens to prepare for the implantation of a fertilised egg (embryo). During pregnancy, the endometrium also helps to form the placenta.

There is significant variation in the thickness of the endometrium at different stages of the menstrual cycle:

- During menstruation: 2–4 mm (0.08–0.2 inches)

- Early proliferative phase (days 6–14): 5–7 mm (0.2–0.3 inches)

- Late proliferative pre-ovulatory phase: up to 11 mm (0.4 inches)

- Secretory phase: 7–16 mm (0.3–0.6 inches)

The growth of the endometrial lining is dependent on the quality of blood flow to the uterus as well as the effect of oestrogen in encouraging the lining to develop.

A number of factors can cause a thin uterine lining:

- Low oestrogen levels: For the endometrium to thicken adequately it is reliant on having normal levels of oestrogen.

- Inadequate blood flow: Blood is the vehicle that carries oestrogen (and a myriad of other hormones) to the uterus. There are a variety of reasons blood flow to the uterus may be compromised. They include:

  - Sedentary lifestyle: Sitting at a desk all day will do nothing for blood circulation generally, and especially not for blood circulation in your pelvic cavity. Try the femoral massage (see above) or find a local Tai Chi instructor and ask them to teach you the posture 'brush knee and push'. This opens up the hips and pelvic basin and is ideal for restoring sluggish circulation in this area.

  - Tilted uterus (retroverted uterus): Normally the uterus should tilt forward, but in about 20 per cent of all women, it tilts backward, or to one side. The malposition of the uterus may cause reduced circulation to the uterus by kinking blood vessels. It's the same principle as water flowing through a garden hose – if the hose is bent over on itself, water flow is reduced.

  - Uterine fibroids: Fibroids can compress blood vessels leading into the uterus or in many cases utilise that blood supply for their own needs.

  - Uterine fibroid embolisation: This is a surgical procedure to cut off blood supply to the fibroids. The result of this is that the fibroids are starved of blood and wither away, but if the blood vessels supplying the fibroids also supply the endometrium, it will fail to thicken as it won't receive an adequate blood supply.

- Infection and pelvic inflammatory disease (PID): Chronic or repeated infection can lead to PID, and a build-up of scar tissue can result. It will be difficult for an even layer of endometrial tissue to form on top of this scar tissue.

- Dilation and curettage (D & C): D & C is a surgical procedure to remove the upper layers of the endometrium. If the deeper layer (the basalis) of the endometrium is removed, the endometrium cannot grow back as the foundation it grows from is gone.

- Long-term use of oral contraceptive pills containing progesterone: This has been linked to the thinning of the uterine lining and uterine atrophy (shrinking of the uterus).

From a Chinese medicine perspective, the essential components for success in getting pregnant include unobstructed Blood flow to the organs that are vital to conception, but also abundant, high-quality Blood. Chicken soup is an old reliable in many cultures, and the following recipe is a good one to build Blood.

 CHICKEN SOUP

Ingredients

- 5 large chicken legs (about 600 g or 1½ lbs)
- 1 tbsp soy sauce
- 2 tbsp rice wine (or sherry)
- 2 cloves garlic, grated or finely chopped
- 2 tbsp fresh root ginger, grated or finely chopped
- 1 tsp brown sugar
- 1 tbsp rice vinegar
- 2 tsp red chilli, finely chopped (seeds in or out – your preference)
- 2 tbsp sesame oil
- 150 g (5 oz) cabbage, chopped
- 2 tbsp spring onions (scallions), thinly sliced
- 475 ml (17 fl oz) chicken stock or water

Method

1. Combine the chicken legs, soy sauce, rice wine, garlic, ginger, sugar, vinegar, chilli and 1 tablespoon of sesame oil in a bowl. Put in the fridge for 30 minutes (or overnight).

2. Heat the remaining tablespoon of sesame oil in a large, heavy pot over a medium heat. Add the cabbage and spring onions and sauté until tender.

3. Add the chicken with the marinade mixture and the stock. Bring to the boil before reducing the heat and simmering until the chicken is cooked through. Serve.

Therapeutic qualities

Chicken: Chicken on the bone has a Qi and Blood tonifying action. Traditionally in Asia 'black chickens' (Silkies) would have been used. While the bird itself is fluffy and white, its flesh is black; this breed is prized above all others for making tonic soups; however, any good quality free range chicken will work for this recipe.

Garlic, chilli and ginger: Are all warming in nature and move stagnant Blood. They also help tonify Spleen Qi. Spleen in Chinese medicine subsumes all digestive functions. In recipes that tonify Spleen Qi it can be assumed that the absorptive function of the Small Intestine is also improved.

Sesame oil: Acts as an envoy, guiding the actions of the other ingredients to their target organs.

Vinegar: Acts as an astringent, holding the Blood.

Sugar: A little sugar can act as a Spleen tonic and aid in the production of Blood.

Cabbage: Acts as a Spleen tonic.

Spring onion: Dispels Blood stasis and expels Cold from the interior. Improves Blood circulation in the smaller blood vessels such as those in the pelvis.

PELVIC INFLAMMATORY DISEASE

PID is a general term for an infection that affects the lining of the uterus (endometrius), the fallopian tubes (salpingitis) and/or the ovaries (oophoritis). It is caused primarily by sexually trans-mitted infections that spread up from the uterus to these organs.

Common symptoms

Many episodes of PID go unrecognised, as women often have no symptoms. It is possible for a woman to have PID and be asymptomatic (without symptoms), or for the symptoms to be too mild to notice, which is the main reason it is under-diagnosed.

Women may also have some of these symptoms listed below, but please bear in mind that there are numerous other conditions that can cause them. Symptoms include:

- Lower abdominal tenderness (usually one-sided)
- Fever that comes and goes
- Abnormal discharge from the vagina
- Pain or bleeding during or after intercourse
- Irregular menstrual bleeding
- Spotting between periods
- Period pain
- Pain during ovulation
- Frequent or burning urination
- Swollen abdomen
- Swollen lymph nodes
- Nausea or vomiting
- Pain around the kidneys
- Pain in the upper right portion of the abdomen
- Lower back pain that may radiate down the insides of the legs.

The intensity and extent of the symptoms depends on which micro organisms are causing the problem, where they are located (uterus, tubes, lining of the abdomen, etc.), how long the woman has had PID, what, if any, antibiotics have been taken, and general health.

Complications

Infection within the fallopian tubes is the worst outcome in terms of fertility. The normally smooth inner surface of the fallopian tube can become scarred or totally blocked as a result of chronic infection. This scar tissue blocks or interrupts the normal movement of eggs into the uterus. There are two primary concerns with scarred fallopian tubes:

- If a fertilised egg begins to grow in the tube as if it were in the uterus, the result is an ectopic pregnancy. As it grows, an ectopic pregnancy can rupture the fallopian tube, causing severe pain, internal bleeding and, in some cases, even death.

- If the fallopian tubes are totally blocked by scar tissue, the sperm cannot fertilise an egg, and the woman becomes infertile.

Approximately 15 per cent of women are infertile after a single episode of PID, 25–35 per cent after two episodes and 50–75 per cent after three or more episodes.

Self-help treatment for PID

Due to its complex nature and difficulties in getting a definitive diagnosis, PID is generally not amenable to self-treatment. It may, however, be worth taking grapefruit seed extract (GSE) as a daily supplement. As the study below shows, it is a potent anti-bacterial and anti-fungal agent. If you are taking prescribed medication of any sort, talk to your healthcare practitioner before taking GSE.

> The initial data shows GSE to have antimicrobial properties against a wide range of gram-negative and gram-positive organisms at dilutions found to be safe. With the aid of scanning transmission electron microscopy (STEM), the mechanism of GSE's antibacterial activity was revealed. It was evident that GSE disrupts the bacterial membrane and liberates the cytoplasmic

contents within 15 minutes after contact even at more dilute concentrations. (Heggers *et al.* 2002)

REFERENCES AND FURTHER READING

Broekmans, F. J., Kwee, J., Hendriks, D. J., Mol, B. W. and Lambalk, C. B. (2006) 'A systematic review of tests predicting ovarian reserve and IVF outcome.' *Human Reproduction Update 12*, 685–718.

Chuang, C. C., Chen, C. D., Chao, K. H., Chen, S. U., Ho, H. N. and Yang, Y. (2003) 'Age is a better predictor of pregnancy potential than basal follicle-stimulating hormone levels in women undergoing *in vitro* fertilization.' *Fertility and Sterility 79*, 63–68.

Hale, L. P., Greer, P. K., Trinh, C. T. and James, C. L. (2005) 'Proteinase activity and stability of natural bromelain preparations.' *International Immunopharmacology 5, 4*, 783–793.

Heggers, J. P., Cottingham, J., Gusman, J. *et al.* (2002) 'The effectiveness of processed grapefruit-seed extract as an antibacterial agent. II: Mechanism of action and in vitro toxicity.' *Journal of Alternative and Complementary Medicine 8, 3*, 333–340.

Kaptchuk, T. K. (2000) *Chinese Medicine: The Web that Has No Weaver.* London: Rider, an imprint of Ebury Press, Random House.

Martinez, F. and Lopez-Arregui, E. (2009) 'Infection risk and intrauterine devices.' *Acta Obstetricia et Gynecologica Scandinavica 88, 3*, 246–250.

Mylonas, I. (2012) 'Female genital Chlamydia trachomatis infection: Where are we heading?' *Archives of Gynecology and Obstetrics 285, 5*, 1271–1285.

Nelson, L. M. (2009) 'Primary ovarian insufficiency.' *New England Journal of Medicine 360*, 606–614.

Newell, S. D., Crofts, J. F. and Grant, S. R. (2014) 'The incarcerated gravid uterus: Complications and lessons learned.' *Obstetrics and Gynaecology 12*, 423–427.

Paavonen, J. (2012) 'Chlamydia trachomatis infections of the female genital tract: State of the art.' *Annals of Medicine 44, 1*, 18–28.

Purcell, S. and Moley, K. (2011) 'The impact of obesity on egg quality.' *Journal of Assisted Reproduction and Genetics 28, 6*, 517–524.

Ross, J. D. (2005) 'Is mycoplasma genitalium a cause of pelvic inflammatory disease?' *Infectious Disease Clinics of North America 19, 2*, 407–413.

Scott, R. T., Toner, J. P., Muasher, S. J., Oehninger, S., Robinson, S. and Rosenwaks, Z. (1989) 'Follicle-stimulating hormone levels on cycle day 3 are predictive of *in vitro* fertilization outcome.' *Fertility and Sterility 51*, 651.

Unschuld, P. U. and Tessenow, H. (2011) *Huang Di Nei Jing Su Wen: An Annotated Translation of Huang Di's Inner Classic – Basic Questions.* Berkeley, CA, and London: University of California Press.

Chapter 8

PERIOD PAIN

Period pain (dysmenorrhoea) is probably the most common gynaecological issue to present in any clinic, be it a Chinese medicine or biomedicine one. According to the International Association for the Study of Pain (2007), up to 90 per cent of women experience menstrual cramps on a regular basis.

Period pain can be divided into primary and secondary dysmenorrhoea. This distinction is important as later onset period pain may be a symptom of an underlying pathology (see below).

PERIOD PAIN IN BIOMEDICINE

Primary dysmenorrhoea

Primary dysmenorrhoea usually occurs around the time that the menstrual cycle begins, and in most cases there will be a well-established pattern of menstrual pain within two years if it is going to occur.

Typical symptoms include:

- Dull aching pain in the abdomen
- Feeling of pressure in the abdomen
- Pain in the lower back and/or inner thighs
- Nausea or vomiting
- Chronic loose stools.

The cause of primary dysmenorrhoea is not understood, but most symptoms can be explained by the action of uterine prostaglandins (a group of compounds that have diverse hormone-like effects in mammals, including humans). The prostaglandins made in the uterus make the uterine muscles contract and shed the lining that has built up over the course of the previous month. If excessive prostaglandins are produced, they can cause the severe muscular cramping that many women will recognise as period pain. Prostaglandins produced in other sites within the body can also cause headaches, nausea, vomiting and diarrhoea.

Secondary dysmenorrhoea

Secondary dysmenorrhoea is pain that is caused by a disorder in a woman's reproductive organs, such as endometriosis, adenomyosis, uterine fibroids or infection (PID). Pain from secondary dysmenorrhoea usually begins earlier in the menstrual cycle and lasts longer than common menstrual cramps. Secondary dysmenorrhoea is much less common than primary dysmen-orrhoea. It is also more likely to affect you if you are between the ages of 30 and 45. The most likely causes of secondary dysmenorrhoea are:

- Endometriosis: A condition in which the tissue lining the uterus (the endometrium) is found outside of the uterus (see Chapter 5).

- Pelvic inflammatory disease (PID): An infection caused by bacteria that starts in the uterus and can spread to other reproductive organs (see Chapter 7).

- Fibroids: These are non-cancerous growths within, on or pushing out from the wall of the uterus. These often cause pain and very heavy bleeding (see Chapter 6).

- Adenomyosis: This is a growth of the uterine lining into the wall of the uterus. This condition is associated with endometriosis and is more likely to affect you if you have already had a baby.

- Cervical stenosis: A narrowing of the opening to the uterus.

PERIOD PAIN IN CHINESE MEDICINE

Effective treatment strategies for menstrual pain have existed for centuries, and some from *Furen Liangfang Jiyao* (*The Complete Dictionary of Effective Prescriptions for Women*) (published in 1237 AD) are still as effective today as during the Three Kingdoms period (Dynasty) (220–280 AD).

COMMON SYMPTOMS

- Pain: In general it can be argued that there are two basic patterns that are the cause of most period pain:

  - Qi stagnation, a dull achy pain that responds to movement (things like rubbing your back or abdomen). Other symptoms common with this pattern include emotional instability, angry thoughts or outbursts, sensations of being too warm or actually running a temperature, and abdominal and/or breast distension. A hot water bottle or a gentle massage gives relief from the symptoms.

  - Blood stagnation, a sharp stabbing pain that is fixed in location and does not come and go. The pain can become more severe in nature in the days leading up to and the first 24 hours of a period. Blood clots will be common with a period. Over-the-counter or prescribed medication is needed for pain relief.

- Heat: Frustration, angry outbursts, red flushed face and elevated temperature and headaches pre period can all be symptoms of excess Heat (normally due to Qi stagnation and a lack of free movement). A small rise in temperature is normal after ovulation as progesterone levels increase, but for symptoms to occur, something pathological is occurring.

- Abdominal and/or breast distension: These are typical symptoms of Qi stagnation. Belching, flatulence or hiccupping are also likely.

- Deficiency: The Blood loss at a period is obvious, but you also lose Qi, as Qi moves Blood. A lot of post-period symptoms such as dizziness, fatigue, headaches, insomnia or poor coordination are due to Qi and/or Blood deficiency.

VITAMIN AND MINERAL SUPPLEMENTS

Vitamin B6: Plays a key role in the synthesis of the neurotransmitter dopamine, which is thought to promote physical and emotional wellbeing. Clinical studies have shown that vitamin B6 can reduce pain levels. Researchers are not sure whether the painkilling effect is due to some unknown chemical mechanism or just the fact that vitamin B6 makes people feel better (see Guilarte 1989).

Vitamin D: Recent Danish research (see Deutch 1995) has shown that women with relatively low vitamin D levels (less than 45 nanograms per millilitre (ng/mL)) who took a 300,000 IU mega-dose of vitamin D3 had a significant reduction in menstrual cramp pain.

Vitamin E: Taking vitamin E a few days prior to the onset of and during menstruation has been shown to significantly reduce menstrual pain as well as to limit the amount of blood lost during menstruation.

Calcium: A number of scientific studies suggest that an increased intake of calcium can alleviate menstrual cramps (see Penland and Johnson 1993). The exact mechanisms by which calcium decreases cramps are not fully understood, but researchers suspect that it is related to the role of this important mineral in maintaining normal muscle tone. Calcium-deficient muscles are more likely to be tense, which may trigger menstrual cramps. Getting the balance right here is critical as excessive amounts of calcium can cause muscles to become tense.

Magnesium: Magnesium supplements have been found to reduce the symptoms of period pain in clinical studies. The reason for this is most likely that magnesium is a very effective muscle relaxant, and most menstrual pain can, to a greater or smaller degree, be attributed to a spasm in the muscle walls of the uterus.

Omega-3 fatty acids: Diets low in omega-3 fatty acids have been associated with menstrual pain. In a recent double-blind trial, supplementation with fish oil, a good source of omega-3 fatty acids, led to a 37 per cent drop in menstrual symptoms (see Kheirkhah *et al.* 2016).

Zinc: Zinc supplements a few days prior to the onset of menses have been shown to prevent premenstrual pain and bloating.

THERAPEUTIC RECIPES

For a complete listing of the energetic qualities and uses in Chinese medicine of most common foods, see Appendix A.

The aim with all the recipes below is to move Qi and Blood, which will prevent stagnation. You are not limited to just the recipes below, however; in general, any mildly spicy dishes such as a mild curry or a stir-fry with aromatic vegetables (onions, peppers, chilli, spring onions) or spices (ginger, galangal, turmeric) will work. The aim is to keep things moving all month, not just around a period – don't wait until you have symptoms to take action. For severe period pain try some of the recipes listed for endometriosis in Chapter 5.

Breakfast

Porridge made with water and sprinkled with cinnamon. Porridge is warming in nature; it improves digestive function and Blood circulation. Cinnamon improves Blood circulation in the smaller vessels such as those in the fingers, toes or around the reproductive organs.

Walnuts and/or cashews in natural yoghurt. Although yoghurt is considered cold in nature, both walnuts and cashews are warming. It is important to choose yoghurt with no added sugar and live bacteria.

Lunch

Salad: Many salad vegetables are cold in nature (this can slow down digestive function and impair the movement of Qi and Blood), but the addition of onions, garlic, ginger, chilli or peppers can mediate the cooling action of the vegetables.

Try some of the following combinations:

Carrot, apple and ginger

Carrot and radish

Duck, watercress and orange

Guacamole

Mixed beans with chilli

Prawns with bean sprouts

Dinner

 GINGER BROCCOLI

Ingredients

- 1 tbsp sunflower oil
- 1 garlic clove, grated or finely chopped
- 1 tsp fresh root ginger, grated or finely chopped
- 60 g (2 oz) broccoli (or 2 large florets)
- 1 tbsp soy sauce
- 1 tbsp rice vinegar

Method

1. Heat the oil in a large pan over a medium heat.

2. Add the garlic and ginger and cook until fragrant but not browned (about 30 seconds).

3. Add the broccoli and cook, stirring, until the broccoli is bright green.

4. Drizzle a few spoons of water over the broccoli, add the soy sauce, reduce the heat, cover and cook until the broccoli is just tender.

5. Stir in the rice vinegar and serve.

Therapeutic qualities

Broccoli: Acts as a Blood tonic; its cool, sweet nature has a calming influence.

Ginger and garlic: Their warm aromatic nature balances the cool, sweet nature of the broccoli; they also gently move Qi and Blood and prevent stagnation.

Sunflower oil: Thermally neutral.

Soy sauce: Dispels Empty Heat that has resulted from any lack of free movement (stagnation = symptoms).

GINGER FISH

Ingredients

- sea salt
- 2 mackerel fillets
- 2 cm ($\frac{4}{5}$ inch) fresh root ginger, grated or finely chopped
- zest of 1 orange
- 2 spring onions (scallions), finely sliced
- 2 tbsp soy sauce
- 1 tbsp sesame oil
- 1 tbsp olive oil

Method

1. Rub the sea salt all over the mackerel fillets.
2. Put the grated ginger and orange zest on a plate with the fillets on top, skin side up.
3. Steam the fish for 5 minutes.
4. Scatter the spring onions over the fish, then drizzle with the soy sauce.
5. Heat the sesame oil with the olive oil until smoking hot, then pour it over the fish and serve.

Therapeutic qualities

Mackerel: Their sweet nature acts to harmonise as well as tonify Blood.

Ginger, orange zest and spring onions: They all have a warm, aromatic nature that gently disperses Qi stagnation.

Olive oil: Is thermally neutral, and is just a cooking medium.

Sesame oil and sea salt: Envoy to the Kidney Channel.

 ## PORK HOCK IN SOY SAUCE

Ingredients

- 1 medium onion, finely chopped
- 1 tbsp coconut oil
- 2 cloves garlic, crushed
- 1 pork hock (available from your butcher)
- 60 ml (2 fl oz) rice vinegar
- 60 ml (2 fl oz) soy sauce
- 60 ml (2 fl oz) rice wine (or sherry)
- handful of wood ear mushrooms (available in any Asian supermarket)
- 1 tsp five spice powder (see page 67)

Method

1. Sweat the onion in a pot with the coconut oil and garlic.

2. Add the rest of the ingredients, bring to the boil and simmer for 2 hours.

3. Remove and de-bone the pork hock before stirring the meat back into the soup. Serve.

Therapeutic qualities

Pork hock: Nourishes Kidney Yin and Blood.

Rice vinegar: Breaks Blood stasis and stops bleeding (Blood can build up behind a clot until the pressure causes a rupture).

Rice wine: Moves Qi and Blood.

Coconut oil: Nourishes Yin as it moves Qi and Blood.

Wood ear mushrooms: Break Blood stasis.

Onion and garlic: Their aromatic nature prevents the soup from becoming too cloying (too many Yin tonics can lead to Dampness/oedema).

Five spice powder: Cinnamon moves Qi and Blood in the smaller vessels, cloves break Blood stasis, Szechuan peppercorns tonify Qi, fennel seeds envoy to the lower Jiao and star anise tonifies Qi.

LAMB WITH SPRING ONIONS

Ingredients

- 2 tbsp soy sauce
- sea salt
- 1 tbsp rice wine (or sherry)
- 2 tbsp olive oil
- 200 g (7 oz) lean lamb, finely sliced
- 1 tbsp vinegar
- 1 tbsp sesame oil
- 2 tsp ground Szechuan peppercorns or black peppercorns
- 2 garlic cloves, grated or finely chopped
- 2 spring onions (scallions), sliced

Method

1. Mix together 1 tbsp of the soy sauce, some salt, rice wine and the oil. Add the lamb slices and leave to marinate. Mix the remaining soy sauce with the vinegar, sesame oil and peppercorns in a small bowl.

2. Heat the remaining oil in the pan. Add the garlic and stir-fry for 10 seconds. Add the lamb and stir-fry until browned.

3. Garnish with the spring onions and serve.

Therapeutic qualities

Lamb: Qi tonic. Many women find their energy levels drop during a period – tonifying Qi and Blood should help prevent this dip.

Garlic: Moves Blood and prevents clotting. Severe stabbing period pain is often a symptom of Blood stasis.

Szechuan peppercorns and spring onions: Move Qi, reinforcing the action of the garlic. If Qi is moving freely, it keeps Blood moving and stops stagnation.

Rice wine: Moves Qi and Blood, reinforcing the action of the foods above.

Vinegar: Clears Heat (inflammation). Its astringent nature prevents reckless movement of Qi or Blood, and keeps everything in its proper place.

Soy sauce: Dispels Empty Heat that has resulted from any lack of free movement (stagnation = symptoms).

ASPARAGUS IN GINGER SAUCE

Ingredients

- 6 spears of asparagus
- 300 ml (10 fl oz) chicken or vegetable stock
- 2 tbsp soy sauce
- 1 tsp brown sugar
- 1 tbsp rice wine (or dry sherry)
- 1 tbsp vegetable oil
- 2 tsp fresh root ginger, grated or finely chopped
- 1 spring onion (scallion), finely chopped

Method

1. Trim the woody ends off the asparagus and cut the stalks diagonally into 5 cm (2 inch) pieces.

2. In a bowl mix the stock, soy sauce, sugar and rice wine.

3. Heat the oil in a wok or frying pan, add the ginger and spring onion, and stir-fry for 10 seconds. Add the asparagus and stir-fry for a few seconds more.

4. Add the stock mixture to the wok and bring to a boil. Cover and simmer until the asparagus is tender. Serve.

Therapeutic qualities

Asparagus: Clears Heat and promotes Blood circulation in the pelvic region. Asparagus has a special affinity with the Kidneys and urinary tract, and it strongly envoys to this area.

Soy sauce: Dispels Empty Heat that has resulted from any lack of free movement (stagnation = symptoms).

Sugar: Its sweet nature harmonises the Earth element. Comfort eating around the time of a period can be an indication of an imbalance in this element.

Ginger and spring onions: Move Qi and Blood. Due to the affinity of asparagus for the Kidneys and urinary tract, the focus of Qi and Blood movement will be in these areas.

Rice wine: Moves Qi and Blood, reinforcing the action of the ginger and spring onions.

AROMATIC PORK CHOPS

Ingredients

- 3 tbsp soy sauce
- 3 tbsp sesame oil
- 3 tbsp rice wine (or sherry)
- 1 clove garlic, grated or finely chopped
- 2 tsp fresh root ginger, grated or finely chopped
- 1 shallot (or onion), finely chopped
- sea salt
- pork chops
- 2 tbsp honey
- 2 tbsp sesame oil

Method

1. Combine the soy sauce, 3 tbsp sesame oil, rice wine, garlic, ginger, shallot and salt in a large bowl, add the pork chops and coat in the mixture. Marinate for up to 24 hours.

2. Combine the honey and 2 tbsp sesame oil in a small bowl.

3. Heat the sesame oil and honey in a frying pan, add the marinated pork chops and baste them with the honey mixture as they cook. Serve.

Therapeutic qualities

Garlic and ginger: Move Blood and prevent clotting. Severe stabbing period pain is often a symptom of Blood stasis.

Shallots: Move Qi, reinforcing the action of the spices above. If Qi is moving freely, it keeps Blood moving and stops stagnation.

Rice wine: Moves Qi and Blood, reinforcing the actions of the foods above.

Pork and honey: Nourish Yin and Blood. Tonifying Blood can help prevent Blood deficiency symptoms such as dizziness, post-period headaches or fatigue.

STIR-FRIED NOODLES

Ingredients

- 150 g (5 oz) noodles
- 60 g (2 oz) broccoli (or 2 florets), cut into bite-size pieces
- 1 carrot, cut into bite-size pieces
- 3 tbsp olive oil

- 1 onion, finely chopped
- 2 spring onions (scallions), finely sliced
- 2 tsp fresh root ginger, grated or finely chopped
- 3 tbsp soy sauce
- 1 tbsp sesame oil

Method

1. Cook the noodles in boiling salted water. About 2 minutes from the noodles being ready, add the broccoli and carrot.

2. Heat the olive oil in a wok or frying pan, add the onion, spring onions and ginger and stir-fry for 30 seconds.

3. Add the noodles, soy sauce and sesame oil.

4. Mix all the ingredients thoroughly and serve.

Therapeutic qualities

Noodles: The nature of the noodles will vary with the ingredients (see Appendix A).

Ginger and onion: Move Qi and Blood to prevent stagnation.

Soy sauce: Dispels Empty Heat that has resulted from any lack of free movement (stagnation = symptoms).

Olive oil: Is thermally neutral.

Sesame oil: Kidney Qi tonic. The Kidneys have a controlling function on all aspects of the menstrual cycle.

Broccoli and carrot: Blood tonics. Tonifying Blood can help prevent Blood deficiency symptoms such as dizziness, post-period headaches or fatigue.

BEEF CURRY

Ingredients (for 2 portions)

- 2 tbsp olive oil
- 2 bay leaves
- 2 tsp ground cloves
- 4 cardamom pods
- 3 tsp ground cinnamon
- 1 onion, finely chopped
- 2 tsp fresh root ginger, grated or finely chopped
- 2 cloves garlic, grated or finely chopped
- 250 g (9 oz) beef, chopped into pieces
- 2 tsp ground coriander
- 2 tsp chilli powder
- 2 tsp ground turmeric
- sea salt
- 470 ml (17 fl oz) water

Method

1. Heat the oil in a heavy-bottomed pan and add the bay leaves, cloves, cardamom pods, cinnamon and chopped onion and fry until the onions are translucent.

2. Add the ginger and garlic and fry for 30 seconds.

3. Add the beef and other spices and water, and mix everything well.

4. Cook until the meat is tender and the sauce has thickened. Add sea salt to taste and serve.

Therapeutic qualities

Beef: Qi and Blood tonic. Tonifying QI and Blood can help prevent deficiency symptoms such as fatigue, dizziness, post-period headaches or insomnia.

Cloves, turmeric, cinnamon and garlic: Move Blood and prevent clotting. Severe stabbing period pain is often a symptom of Blood stasis.

Ginger, chilli and onion: Move Qi, reinforcing the action of the spices above. If Qi is moving freely, it keeps Blood moving and stops stagnation.

Cardamom: Stops bloating and nausea by promoting proper Qi flow.

Coriander: Regulates Qi flow. If Qi is moving as it should be, there will be a dramatic reduction in symptoms.

PAPAYA SALAD

Ingredients

- 1 papaya
- 1 clove garlic, grated or finely chopped
- 1 red chilli, finely sliced
- 2 tbsp soy sauce
- 2 tbsp vegetable oil (not olive oil – sunflower oil works well)
- 3 tbsp lime juice
- 2 tbsp brown sugar
- 40 g (2 oz) cherry tomatoes, halved
- 40 g (2 oz) bean sprouts
- 50 g (2 oz) walnuts
- 3 spring onions (scallions), finely sliced
- handful of fresh basil, chopped

Method

1. Peel the papaya, then grate it, rotating it as you go to avoid hitting the inner seeds.

2. If you have a food processor add the garlic, chilli, soy sauce, oil, lime juice and brown sugar and pulse until the liquid turns reddish from the chilli. If you don't have a food processor, grate all the ingredients finely, add the sugar and soy sauce, and stir well.

3. Put the papaya in a large bowl, pour over the dressing and toss; add the tomatoes, bean sprouts, walnuts, spring onions and basil, toss again and serve.

Therapeutic qualities

Papaya: Increases Qi and Blood flow in breast tissue and is particularly useful in helping prevent menstrual breast pain or tenderness. Papaya contains enzymes (chymopapain and papain) that break down proteins such as blood clots (note that eating papaya may temporarily cause heavier periods, but with less pain).

Chilli, garlic and spring onion: Move Qi and Blood, preventing stagnation. The chilli and walnuts mediate the cooling action of the papaya, tomato, soy sauce, bean sprouts and lime juice.

Soy sauce: Clears Heat.

Brown sugar: Its sweet nature harmonises the Earth element. Comfort eating around the time of a period can be an indication of an imbalance in this element.

Lime juice: Without the astringent lime juice to counteract the Blood-moving qualities of the papaya, chilli, garlic and spring onion, there could be heavier than normal menstrual bleeding.

Walnuts: Tonify Qi and Blood.

Bean sprouts: Clear Heat.

Tomatoes: Clear Heat and produce Body Fluids. Body Fluids are an integral part of Blood, and ensuring adequate reserves at the time of a period ensures symptoms of Blood deficiency can be avoided post-period.

 ## BEEF AND GINGER CASSEROLE

Ingredients

- 2 tbsp sesame oil
- 1 clove garlic, grated or finely chopped
- 1 onion, finely sliced
- 150 g (5 oz) braising steak, cut into bite-size pieces
- 100 g (3½ oz) button mushrooms
- 1 carrot, sliced
- 2 tsp fresh root ginger, grated or finely chopped
- 1 tbsp soy sauce
- 1 tbsp honey
- 200 ml (7 fl oz) beef stock
- sea salt and black pepper

Method

1. Heat the sesame oil in a casserole dish or large pot, gently cook the garlic and onion, add the beef and allow it to brown.

2. Add all the rest of the ingredients, and cook for 2 hours on a medium heat. Serve.

Therapeutic qualities

Beef: Qi and Blood tonic. It is important to replace what is lost during a period.

Mushrooms: Clear Heat. A lack of free movement can cause sensations of excessively elevated temperature as well as contributing to emotional volatility.

Carrots and honey: Nourish Yin and Blood. It is important to replace what is lost during a period.

Soy sauce: Clears Heat.

Onions and ginger: Move Qi and Blood. The warm nature of the onion and ginger mediates the cooling qualities of the soy sauce, carrots, mushrooms and honey.

ACUPRESSURE

How to apply pressure to the points

To press points, use something blunt. You can use finger pressure, but if you have to apply sustained pressure, you may find it uncomfortable. A chopstick (like the ones you get with a takeaway meal) is ideal for this purpose.

Ideally have someone do the treatment for you; that way you are not creating muscular tension while you try and reach points. You can also focus more on what sensations (or lack of them) result from pressing the point.

Don't press too hard; use enough pressure that you (or your partner) can feel something happening.

When you get to the point where something is happening, keep the pressure constant and hold for 30 seconds.

If you are not feeling any effects from pressing a point, you may not be pressing on the exact right spot. Try different spots around the location you first tried.

The points

There are any number of points that can be used, and in most cases points used in an acupuncture treatment are selected based on signs and symptoms presenting at that time. The points listed below are all useful in the treatment of period pain, but for a more individualised treatment plan, talk to a licensed acupuncture practitioner.

LIVER 1 (DA DUN) GREAT ESTEEM

Actions – Regulates Qi in the genital region, calms the mind.

Location – At the corner of the nail on the inside edge of the big toe.

LIVER 4 (ZHONG FENG) MIDDLE SEAL

Actions – Moves Liver Qi, clears Liver Channel of stagnant Heat.

Location – Find the round bone (medial malleolus) on your inner ankle. Draw an imaginary line from the front of the bone straight down and another line from the bottom of the bone straight across. The point is where the lines intersect.

LIVER 14 (QI MEN) CYCLE GATE

Actions – Moves and regulates Qi, invigorates Blood and disperses masses.

Location – Directly below the nipple in the sixth intercostal space four finger breadths lateral to the breast bone (sternum). If there is Qi stagnation, this point is often very tender and easy to locate.

STOMACH 36 (ZU SAN LI) LEG THREE LI

Actions – Harmonises the Stomach and resolves dampness, tonifies Qi, nourishes Blood and calms the mind.

Location – Four finger breadths below the lower border of your kneecap one finger breadth from the outside border of your shin bone.

LARGE INTESTINE 10 (SHOU SAN LI) ARM THREE LI

Actions – Regulates Qi and Blood flow, harmonises the Intestines and Stomach.

Location – On the line joining the cubital crease (the crease that's created when you bend your elbow) and the base of the thumb two finger breadths below the cubital crease.

BLADDER 32 (CI LIAO) SECOND BONE HOLE

Actions – Regulates menstruation.

Location – Over the second sacral foramen (the two dimples in your lower back at the base of your spine).

REN 4 (GUAN YUAN) ORIGIN PASS

Actions – Tonifies and nourishes the Kidneys, benefits the uterus, regulates the Bladder and regulates Small Intestine Qi.

Location – On the anterior midline four finger breadths below the umbilicus.

REFERENCES AND FURTHER READING

Deutch, B. (1995) 'Menstrual pain in Danish women correlated with low n-3 polyunsaturated fatty acid intake.' *European Journal of Clinical Nutrition 49*, 7, 508–516.

Fraser, I. (1992) 'Prostaglandins, prostaglandin inhibitors and their roles in gynaecological disorders.' *Bailliere's Clinical Obstetrics and Gynaecology 6*, 829–857.

Guilarte, T. R. (1989) 'Effect of vitamin B-6 nutrition on the levels of dopamine, dopamine metabolites, dopa decarboxylase activity, tyrosine, and GABA in the developing rat corpus striatum.' *Neurochemical Research 14*, 6, 571–578.

Harlow, S. D. and Campbell, O. M. (2004) 'Epidemiology of menstrual disorders in developing countries: A systematic review.' *BJOG: An International Journal of Obstetrics & Gynaecology 111*, 6–16.

Harlow, S. D. and Park, M. (1996) 'A longitudinal study of risk factors for the occurrence, duration and severity of menstrual cramps in a cohort of college women.' *British Journal of Obstetrics and Gynaecology 103*, 1134–1142.

International Association for the Study of Pain (2007) 'Epidemiology of pain in women.' *Global Year Against Pain in Women: Real Women, Real Pain.* Available at www.iasp-pain.org/files/Content/ContentFolders/GlobalYearAgainstPain2/RealWomenRealPainFactSheets/All_English.pdf

Kheirkhah, M., Gholami, R., Ghare-Shiran, S. Y. and Abbasinia, H. (2016) 'Comparison of the effect of omega-3 fatty acids and perforan (*Hypericum perforatum*) on severity of premenstrual syndrome (PMS): A randomized trial.' *International Journal of Medical Research & Health Sciences 5*, 11, 333–340.

Kirchon, B. and Poindexter, A. N. (1988) 'Contraception: A risk factor for endometriosis.' *Obstetrics & Gynaecology 71*, 6, 829–831.

Lu, Y. (2014) 'Therapeutic observation of triple acupuncture at Zhongji (CV 3) plus mild moxibustion for primary dysmenorrhea.' *Shanghai Journal of Acupuncture and Moxibustion 33*, 7.

Pan, J.-C., Tsai, Y.-T., Lai, J.-N., Fang, R.-C. and Yeh, C.-H. (2014) 'The traditional Chinese medicine prescription pattern of patients with primary dysmenorrhea in Taiwan: A largescale cross sectional survey.' *Journal of Ethnopharmacology 152*, 2, 314–319.

Parazzini, F., Di Cintio, E., Chatenoud, L., Moroni, S., Mezzanotte, C. and Crosanani, P. G. (1999) 'Oral contraceptives – use and risk with endometriosis – Italian Endometriosis Study Group.' *British Journal of Obstetrics 106*, 7, 695–699.

Penland, J. G. and Johnson, P. E. (1993) 'Dietary calcium and manganese effects on menstrual cycle symptoms.' *American Journal of Obstetrics and Gynecology 168*, 5, 1417–1423.

Shen, A.-Y., Wang, T.-S., Huang, M.-H., Liao, C.-H., Chen, S.-J. and Lin, C.-C. (2005) 'Antioxidant and antiplatelet effects of dang-gui-shao-yao-san on human blood cells.' *The American Journal of Chinese Medicine 33*, 5, 747–758.

Sundell, G., Milson, I. and Andersch, B. (1990) 'Factors influencing the prevalence and severity of dysmenorrhoea in young women.' *British Journal of Obstetrics and Gynaecology 97*, 588–594.

Zeraati, F., Shobeiri, F., Nazari, M., Araghchian, M. and Bekhradi, R. (2014) 'Comparative evaluation of the efficacy of herbal drugs (fennelin and vitagnus) and mefenamic acid in the treatment of primary dysmenorrhea.' *Iranian Journal of Nursing and Midwifery Research 19*, 6, 581–584.

Zhao, N. X., Guo, R. L., Ren, Q. Y. *et al.* (2007) 'Acupuncture therapy in treating primary dysmenorrhea, treatment efficacy and hemorheology study.' *Zhejiang University of TCM Journal 31*, 3, 364–365, 367.

Zhou, J. (2014) 'Acupuncture and moxibustion plus herbal hot compress for primary dysmenorrhea.' *Journal of Clinical Acupuncture and Moxibustion 60*, 2, 11–13.

Zondervan, K. T., Yudkin, P. L., Vessey, M. P. *et al.* (1998) 'The prevalence of chronic pelvic pain in the United Kingdom: A systematic review.' *British Journal of Obstetrics and Gynaecology 105*, 93–99.

Chapter 9

PELVIC PAIN

Pelvic pain can be the result of many different factors. In some cases there is a specific disorder that causes or exacerbates symptoms, while in other cases the cause is unknown.

Pelvic pain can range from sudden acute attacks to recurrent attacks of pain that may or may not be related to a woman's menstrual cycle, to chronic persistent pain that lasts weeks or months.

In many cases biomedicine can find no cause for pelvic pain, even in cases where there is an underlying previously diagnosed pathology; for example, chronic pelvic pain often coexists with endometriosis, but the endometriosis is not seen as the root cause of the pain.

COMMON CONDITIONS THAT
CAN CAUSE PELVIC PAIN

Many of these conditions have a specific chapter dedicated to them in this book as they need to be explored in more detail. The conditions listed below are included in this chapter as they are likely causes of pelvic pain.

- Endometriosis: A condition in which the lining of the uterus colonises areas outside of the uterus. This tissue continues to be influenced by the hormones that regulate the menstrual cycle and continue to grow in size throughout the month and then cause bleeding at the site of these tissue deposits at the time of a period. This blood has no escape route from the body and it is the resulting build-up of blood and tissue that typically cause the pain associated with endometriosis (see also Chapter 5).

- Pelvic inflammatory disease (PID): This is inflammation of the female genital tract that can be caused by various bacteria as well as internal factors. It can be accompanied by pelvic and lower abdominal pain.

- Interstitial cystitis: This is a condition characterised by lower abdomen or pelvic pain on urination, increased frequency of urination, a sensation that there is always some urine that has not been expressed or a feeling of pressure in the area around the bladder. Unlike 'normal' cystitis, interstitial cystitis tends not to respond to antibiotic treatment, and is in most cases a chronic issue.

- Ovarian cysts: These are a common cause of pelvic pain. In many cases pain and tenderness due to an ovarian cyst will be more pronounced on one side of the abdomen or pelvis. Cysts can range in size from something smaller than a pea to as large as an apple.

- Inflammatory bowel disorders: Conditions such as colitis, diverticulitis and Crohn's disease can be the root cause of pelvic pain. The pain caused by bowel disorders is often experienced as deep recurrent pelvic pain, that may correspond to acute episodes of bowel disease.

- Previous abdominal surgery: Following abdominal surgery it is possible to have adhesions or scar tissue formation between adjacent tissues. It is common that these adhesions can cause pain with certain activities; for example, moving or bending a certain way causes pain.

- Cancers: Cancers of the reproductive and urinary system may cause pain depending on the size of the tumour and the area affected.

SELF-HELP TREATMENTS FOR DEALING WITH PELVIC PAIN

Femoral massage

This massage increases the blood flow to your pelvic organs. This increased blood flow may be useful in clearing any stagnations in the pelvic region (many acupuncture or herbal treatments will be trying to accomplish the same thing, albeit a bit more forcefully).

Locating your femoral artery

The femoral artery is located level with your pubic bone, just beneath the crease in your groin between your thigh and lower abdomen.

How to do it

Compress the femoral artery with your fingers – fairly heavy pressure will be required. When you feel the flow has ceased, hold for 30 seconds. The blood will then back up and increase the pressure in the iliac arteries which forces more blood into the pelvic arteries. This floods the pelvic organs with more blood. When the hold is released, you should feel a sensation of warmth rushing down your legs as the blood supply returns to the lower extremities.

Contraindications

Do not perform this exercise if you are pregnant, have high blood pressure, have heart disease or circulatory problems (aneurisms, varicose veins, phlebitis, thrombosis), have a history of strokes or detached retinas.

Magnesium sulphate (Epsom Salts) foot soaks

A major cause of pain is the excessive stimulation of a protein called NMDA (N-methyl-D-aspartate). The medications normally used to prevent excessive stimulation of NMDA cause significant negative side effects. Magnesium seems to balance NMDA levels without the toxicity (see Rondón *et al.* 2010).

For home use the easiest way to make use of the painkilling properties of magnesium sulphate is to soak your feet in it. Certain substances can be absorbed by the body via the skin very easily (trans-dermal absorption), and magnesium is one of them. Try soaking your feet in a basin with Epsom Salts and warm water.

Castor oil packs

Castor oil contains a unique fatty acid (ricinoleic acid) that is anti-bacterial, anti-fungal and anti-viral, and it may well be worth using in cases of PID or interstitial cystitis as an adjunct treatment to antibiotics.

What you need

- 100–300 ml (3.4–10 fl oz) castor oil
- a cloth (slightly damp)
- cling film (plastic wrap)
- towel
- hot water bottle.

Method

Heat the castor oil in a saucepan, then pour on to the cloth. Apply the cloth (oil side against the skin) over the lower abdominal area. Wrap with cling film and cover with a towel and hot water bottle. Lie down and relax for a while (15–30 minutes) before removing and washing off the oil.

Contraindications

Do not use castor oil packs if you are pregnant.

Mustard and turmeric poultice

A mustard poultice can be very effective in cases where over-the-counter heat patches help to soothe pain in conditions such as endometriosis. Turmeric is a potent anti-inflammatory; it helps to relieve pain and promotes healing. Caution: Mustard can 'burn' skin if it is in direct contact with it. To avoid this, wrap the poultice in a couple of layers of muslin or a face cloth before applying.

DIETARY CONSIDERATIONS

The average Western diet includes far too many foods rich in omega-6 fatty acids, and far too few rich in omega-3 fatty acids. In cases where the normal ratio of omega-3 and 6 fatty acids are altered, inflammatory conditions can develop, as omega-6 fatty acids in excess can promote inflammation. This inflammation can often be of a chronic nature (often referred to as low-grade systemic inflammation) and unrelated to a specific named condition.

Try taking a high-quality cold-pressed fish oil (ask your pharmacist or health food shop).

VITAMIN AND MINERAL SUPPLEMENTS

Your pelvis is composed of a number of bones joined by ligaments and separated by cartilage (fibrous pads that prevent the bones rubbing off each other).

The supplements listed below should help with pain of the bones, caused by either ligament or cartilage damage rather than pain caused by structures within your pelvis; for example, endothelial lesions deep inside your pelvis causing pain to radiate outward.

Chondroitin sulfate and glucosamine: Naturally occurring substances manufactured from sugar proteins, both are important components of cartilage. Go into any health food shop and ask them about remedies for joint pain, and this combination is likely to be the first thing recommended, and with good reason – it can be effective.

Vitamin B3 (Niacin): Acts as an anti-inflammatory by improving micro-circulation within the joint.

Vitamin C: Important for the structural integrity of bones, ligaments and tendons as well as playing a key role in the formation of collagen (a major component of cartilage and bone).

Vitamin D: Helps reduce inflammation.

Vitamin E: Also required for both the formation and maintenance of healthy cartilage.

Vitamin K: Deficiency can result in abnormal cartilage and bone mineralisation.

Copper: Increases joint flexibility, supports bone and connective tissue growth and reduces joint inflammation. It also plays a vital role in stimulating the binding of collagen and elastin.

Manganese: Plays a major role in the formation of cartilage.

Selenium: Acts as an anti-inflammatory.

Sodium: Contributes to the formation of cartilage.

THERAPEUTIC RECIPES

For a complete listing of the energetic qualities and uses in Chinese medicine of most common foods, see Appendix A.

Inflammation (Heat) or infection (Damp Heat) are the most likely root causes in chronic pelvic pain. The recipes below are all focused on clearing inflammation and providing cartilage and bone with the nutrients needed for repair and regeneration.

Breakfast

Porridge made with water and sprinkled with cinnamon. Porridge is warming in nature; it improves digestive function and Blood circulation. Cinnamon improves Blood circulation in the smaller vessels such as those in the fingers, toes or around the reproductive organs.

Walnuts and/or cashews in natural yoghurt. Although yoghurt is considered cold in nature, both walnuts and cashews are warming. It is important to choose yoghurt with no added sugar and live bacteria.

Lunch

Salad: Many salad vegetables are cold in nature (this can slow down digestive function and impair the movement of Qi and Blood), but the addition of onions, garlic, ginger, chilli or peppers can mediate the cooling action of the vegetables.

Try some of the following combinations:

Carrot, apple and ginger

Carrot and radish

Duck, watercress and orange

Guacamole

Mixed beans with chilli

Prawns with bean sprouts

Dinner

GARLIC PEPPER AND PORK RIBS SOUP

Ingredients

- 4 tsp Szechuan peppercorns
- 1 bulb garlic
- 180 g (7 oz) pork ribs
- sea salt

Method

1. Put all the ingredients in a stock pot with 2 litres (8½ cups) of water. Bring to a boil, remove any foam and reduce the heat. Cook on a medium heat for 1 hour.

2. Add sea salt to taste and serve. Drink the soup only.

Therapeutic qualities

Szechuan peppercorns and garlic: Move Qi and Blood.

Pork ribs: Nourish Yin.

GINGER CHICKEN SOUP

Ingredients

- 1 free range chicken, 1–1½ kg (2–3½ lbs)
- 150 g (5 oz) fresh root ginger
- root vegetables of your choice (such as parsnips, carrots, etc.), peeled and chopped into bite-size pieces
- sea salt

Method

1. Remove the chicken skin and cut the chicken into quarters.

2. Peel the ginger and cut it into thick slices.

3. Put all the ingredients into a pot with 2.5 litres (8 cups) of water. Bring to the boil, skim any foam from the soup, reduce the heat and let it simmer for 90 minutes.

4. There is no need to sieve, but for a smoother soup, remove the cooked chicken, blend the ginger and vegetables, and add back in the chicken pieces.

5. Add salt to taste, and serve.

Therapeutic qualities

Chicken: Nourishes Qi and Blood. Cooking the chicken on the bone adds to the soup's ability to nourish connective tissue.

Ginger root: Moves Blood.

OX TENDON AND PEPPER SOUP

Ingredients

- 180 g (6 oz) cow tendon (available from your butcher)
- 60 g (2 oz) black peppercorns

Method

1. Cut the tendon into small pieces (or have your butcher do it).

2. Put the tendon pieces and peppercorns in a pot with 2 litres (8 cups) of water and cook over a medium heat until there is approximately 350 ml (12 fl oz) of soup left.

3. Sieve and drink the soup only. Caution: do not consume this soup if you have high blood pressure.

Therapeutic qualities

Beef tendon: Nourishes Kidney Qi and strengthens connective tissues.

Black peppercorns: Moves Qi and Blood.

WATERMELON AND PORK SOUP

Ingredients

- 1 small watermelon or half a large one
- 2 sticks celery
- 2 dates
- sea salt
- 1 pork hock

Method

1. Peel the watermelon, and put the peel, celery, dates, sea salt and the pork into a pot with 2 litres (8 cups) of water.

2. Cook over a medium heat for 2 hours.

3. Dice the melon flesh, add to the pot and cook for another 30 minutes.

4. Remove the pork hock.

5. There is no need to sieve the soup, but it can be blended for a smoother consistency.

6. Drink the soup with the melon.

Therapeutic qualities

Watermelon: Clears Heat (inflammation) and drains Dampness by promoting urination.

Celery: Clears Heat (inflammation) and drains Dampness by promoting urination.

Pork hock: Nourishes Yin and Blood. Cooking the pork on the bone adds to the soup's ability to nourish connective tissue.

Dates: Nourish Blood.

Sea salt: Envoys to the Kidneys and pelvis.

BARLEY AND BEAN STEW

Ingredients

- 40 g (2 oz) pearl barley
- 1 tbsp olive oil
- 1 small onion, finely chopped
- 1 leek, chopped
- 1 carrot, finely diced
- 1 clove garlic, grated or finely chopped
- 50 ml (2 fl oz) vegetable stock
- 400 g (14 oz) tin black beans, drained and rinsed
- handful green cabbage, finely shredded

Method

1. Place the pearl barley in a saucepan and cover with cold water. Bring to the boil, then simmer for 35 minutes until tender. Rinse under cold running water, drain and set aside.

2. Heat the olive oil in a saucepan and add the onion, leek and carrot and cook for 4–5 minutes. Add the garlic and cook for a further 3 minutes.

3. Pour in the stock and bring to the boil. Reduce the heat and simmer for 10 minutes. Add the black beans, barley and cabbage, and simmer for a further 5 minutes. Serve.

Therapeutic qualities

Black beans: Warm and astringent in nature, tonify Kidney Qi.

Pearl barley: Drains Dampness by promoting urination.

Carrot: Nourishes Yin and clears Heat.

Leek: Qi tonic.

Garlic and onion: Dispel Dampness, move Qi.

Cabbage: Drains Dampness by promoting urination, clears Damp Heat.

STICKY SESAME AND WALNUT BALLS

Ingredients

- 60 g (2 oz) black sesame seeds
- 60 g (2 oz) chopped walnuts
- 4 tbsp honey

Method

1. If the sesame seeds aren't already roasted, toast them by putting them in a frying pan or wok over a medium heat, shaking the pan occasionally. Remove the seeds from the pan so they don't overcook, and let them cool.

2. In a food processor, blend together the sesame seeds, walnuts and 3 tbsp of honey.

3. Roll the mix into balls. If the balls don't stick together at first, add a little more honey and blend the mixture some more.

Therapeutic qualities

Black sesame seeds: Tonify the Kidneys.

Walnuts: Tonify Kidney Qi.

Honey: Its cooling action mediates the warming action of the other ingredients.

BONE BROTH

Ingredients

- 1 kg (2 lb) beef bones (any bones will do, but beef is easy to get in large quantities)
- 50 g (2 oz) goji berries
- 2 tbsp apple cider vinegar
- root vegetables of your choice, peeled and chopped into bite-size pieces

Method

1. Place all the ingredients in a large stock pot and cover with cold water. The water level should cover the bones by 5 cm (2 inches) while still leaving room at the top of the pan.

2. Cover with a lid and bring to the boil. Reduce the heat and simmer, lid on, for at least 12 hours, skimming off any foam.

3. Strain and serve. Bone broth will keep in the fridge for up to a week.

Therapeutic qualities

Beef bones: Nourish Yin and Blood. Everything needed for good bone health is contained in the soup bones.

Goji berries: Nourish Yin.

Apple cider vinegar: Helps the nutrients leach out of the bones into the broth.

ACUPRESSURE

There are multiple points and point combinations that can be used to treat pelvic pain. The acupoints listed below could be considered a good basic treatment protocol. You can use all the points listed below or select individual points; see what works for you.

Some things to bear in mind:

• You don't need to use lots of pressure to get results – in many cases, less is more.

• If you want to use some oil, have a look at Appendix A to see what's most appropriate for the condition you are treating.

• If possible, have someone else stimulate the points for you – some are awkward to reach by yourself.

• In general, start with points on or closest to the body and work outwards.

• Stimulate each point for approximately 1 minute. If you find some points work more effectively in relieving your symptoms, focus your efforts on them.

The points
HEART 7 (SHEN MEN) SPIRIT GATE

This point is worth trying in cases where you are stressed or anxious. I find that in many cases points on the Heart or Small Intestine Channel are useful in the treatment of gynaecological issues as the mind can both adversely influence and be adversely influenced in a wide range of pathologies, and gynaecological ones are no exception.

Actions – Calms the mind.

Location – At the ulnar end of the transverse crease of the wrist, in the depression on the radial side of the tendon of the flexor carpi ulnaris muscle.

Location note – On the wrist crease, on the inside edge of the tendon that moves when you wiggle your little finger.

LIVER 3 (TAI CHONG) GREAT SURGE

Points on the Liver Channel are particularity indicated in gynaecological conditions as both the main external portion of the Channel and a divergent branch strongly influencing the genitalia, both internally and externally.

Actions – Smooths the flow of Qi, nourishes Blood, regulates menstruation and regulates the lower abdominal and pelvic regions.

Location – On the dorsum of the foot in the depression distal to the junction of the first and second metatarsal bones.

Location note – Put your finger on the web between the big and second toe. Move your finger up along the back of the foot and you will run into the junction in the bones.

LIVER 8 (QU QUAN) SPRING AT THE BEND

Actions – Benefits the genitals, invigorates Blood, benefits the uterus and nourishes Blood.

Location – When the knee is flexed, the point is at the medial end of the transverse popliteal crease, posterior to the medial epicondyle of the tibia in the depression of the anterior border of the insertions of the semimembranosus and semitendinosus muscles.

Location note – The point is on the inside of the knee, just above the crease that is formed when the knee is bent.

LIVER 12 (JI MAI) URGENT PULSE

Actions – A useful local point when there is congestion or stagnation in the lower abdominal or pelvic areas.

Location – In the inguinal groove where the pulsation of the femoral artery is palpable approximately three finger breadths lateral to the anterior midline.

Location note – Just off and slightly below the pubic bone. Don't press too hard.

LIVER 14 (QI MEN) CYCLE GATE

Actions – Regulates the flow of Qi and invigorates Blood.

Location – Directly below the nipple in the sixth intercostal space four finger breadths lateral to the breast bone (sternum). If there is Qi stagnation, this point is often very tender and easy to locate.

STOMACH 29 (GUI LAI) THE RETURN

Actions – Regulates menstruation and benefits the genital region.

Location – Two finger breadths lateral to the midline and four finger breadths below the umbilicus.

Location note – Draw a line from the belly button and another across one finger breadth above the top of the pubic bone. Where they intersect is the point.

STOMACH 30 (QI CHONG) GREATER RUSHING

Actions – Moves Qi and Blood in the lower abdominal and pelvic areas.

Location – Five finger breadths below the umbilicus (on the top edge of the pubic bone), two finger breadths lateral to the midline.

Location note – The point is at the top upper edge of the pubic bone.

Caution – Do not apply pressure to this point if you are pregnant, have high blood pressure, have heart disease or circulatory problems (aneurisms, varicose veins, phlebitis, thrombosis), have a history of strokes or detached retinas.

SPLEEN 4 (GONG SUN) YELLOW EMPEROR

Actions – Regulates the uterus and resolves Dampness (excessive discharge), calms the mind.

Location – In the depression distal and inferior to the base of the first metatarsal bone at the junction of the red and white skin.

Location note – Slide your finger backwards from the base of your first toe. There is a natural groove formed by a tendon. The point is approximately halfway along your foot.

SPLEEN 6 (SAN YIN JIAO) THREE YIN INTERSECTION

Actions – Resolves dampness (excessive discharge), regulates menstruation, benefits the genitals, invigorates Blood, activates the Channel and alleviates pain.

Location – Three finger breadths directly above the tip of the medial malleolus posterior to the medial border of the tibia.

Location note – The point is three finger breadths above the ankle, midway between the inside edge of the shin bone and the Achilles tendon.

Caution – This point can induce labour, so do not use if you are pregnant.

REFERENCES AND FURTHER READING

Kavic, S. M. (2002) 'Adhesions and adhesiolysis: The role of laparoscopy.' *Journal of the Society of Laparoendoscopic Surgeons 6*, 2, 99–109.

Lini, R., Yunan, D. and Xiulan, L. (2015) 'Analysis of Chinese medicine acupuncture combined treatment for 90 cases of chronic pelvic inflammatory.' *Medical Innovation of China 17*, 4–7.

Oyama, I. A., Rejba, A., Lukban, J. C. *et al.* (2004) 'Thiele massage as therapeutic intervention for female patients with interstitial cystitis and hightone pelvic floor dysfunction.' *Modified Urology 64*, 5, 862–865.

Rondón, L. J., Privat, A. M., Daulhac, L. *et al.* (2010) 'Magnesium attenuates chronic hypersensitivity and spinal cord NMDA receptor phosphorylation in a rat model of diabetic neuropathic pain.' *The Journal of Physiology 588*, 4205–4215.

Royal College of Obstetricians and Gynaecologists (2005) *Chronic Pelvic Pain: Initial Management*. Greentop Guideline No. 41. London: RCOG Press.

Shen, B. Q., Situ, Y., Huang, J. L. *et al.* (2005) 'A clinical study on the treatment of chronic pelvic inflammation of Qi stagnation with Blood stasis syndrome by Penyangqing capsule.' *Chinese Journal of Integrative Medicine 11*, 249–254.

Wang, X. M. (1989) 'On the therapeutic efficacy of electric acupuncture with moxibustion in 95 cases of chronic pelvic infectious disease (PID).' *Journal of Traditional Chinese Medicine 9*, 21–24.

Witt, C. M., Reinhold, T., Brinkhaus, B., Roll, S., Jena, S. and Willich, S. N. (2008) 'Acupuncture in patients with dysmenorrhea: A randomized study on clinical effectiveness and cost-effectiveness in usual care.' *American Journal of Obstetrics & Gynecology 198*, 166.e1–8.

Zheng, H., Wang, S., Shang, J. *et al.* (1998) 'Study on acupuncture and moxibustion therapy for female urethral syndrome.' *Journal of Traditional Chinese Medicine 18*, 2, 122–127.

Zhou, P., Zeng, Z. H. and Xiang, Y. H. (2014) 'Clinical study on chronic pelvic inflammatory disease with syndrome of Damp-heat and Blood-stasis by Qing-Re Li-Shi Hua-Yu decoction combined with acupuncture therapy.' *World Science and Technology – Modernization of Traditional Chinese Medicine 16*, 12.

• Chapter 10 •

PELVIC PAIN IN PREGNANCY

Pelvic girdle pain is a common complaint among pregnant women worldwide, and estimates of pelvic and back pain among pregnant women range from 24 to 90 per cent. This pain can be truly debilitating, and back pain in pregnancy increases the risk of lower back and pelvic pain in the weeks or months (and in some cases, years) after pregnancy.

Pelvic pain in pregnancy is normally caused by the ligaments that bind the pubic bone (symphysis pubis) to the other pelvic bones becoming softened by a hormone called relaxin, and as a result, the pelvic joints become unstable, causing pain. The condition does not have to be associated with pregnancy, but it often is, as the additional weight of the baby and amniotic fluid combined with the pelvic ligaments softening in preparation for labour cause the pelvic bones to move and become misaligned.

RISK FACTORS FOR PELVIC PAIN IN PREGNANCY

The following factors contribute to the chances of developing pelvic pain during pregnancy:

- Engaging in strenuous activities while pregnant. What you define as strenuous will depend on your fitness levels before you became pregnant. In general, exercise during pregnancy is to be encouraged; just make allowances for your changing centre of gravity and energy levels.

- Multiple pregnancies. The ligament-softening hormone relaxin is produced in every pregnancy, especially in the latter part. Ligaments that have softened in response to the production of relaxin may not be as tight as they were post-pregnancy, and with every pregnancy may become ever more lax. The result of this is that the relatively tiny amounts of relaxin produced in early pregnancy may be enough for already softened ligaments to totally relax and cause shifting of the pelvic bones.

- Expecting a large baby or twins. A large baby or multiple babies can cause considerable extra strain on the pelvic ligaments due simply to gravity. A maternity support belt can be especially useful in these cases.

- Poor posture. In this case the root cause is basically mechanical. Your changing centre of gravity combined with increased pressure on the core muscles can cause muscles (that attach to the bones in your lower back and pelvis via tendons) to become strained.

- The position of the foetus. In the latter stages of pregnancy a baby lying on the sciatic nerve is a common cause of pelvic and/or leg pain. This pain is typically one-sided and comes and goes.

- The health of the connective tissues. Pre-existing diseases affecting the connective tissues may be exacerbated by relaxin. In this case the pain may affect all the joints rather than just the pelvis.

- A history of a fracture or trauma to the pelvis.

COMMON SYMPTOMS

Apart from the lower abdomen and pubic pain and discomfort, symphysis pubis dysfunction (SPD) may also lead to the following symptoms:

- Severe pain that tends to get worse when you lift your legs; for example, going up stairs.

- Pain that gets worse when you lie on your back.

- Pain that worsens when you try to turn over in bed.

- Reduced range of movement of the hip bones. This can cause such difficulty walking that crutches may be required.

- Pain shooting down your buttocks and legs; typically this pain will run from your pubic bone down the inside of your thighs.

- A clicking sound coming from your pelvic area when you walk or move your legs.

- Urinary incontinence.

In very rare instances, one or more of the pelvic joints may become dislocated, causing serious pain in the pelvis, hips, groin and buttock. This condition is known as diastasis symphysis pubis. Total bed rest until after delivery is often the preferred treatment option.

SELF-HELP FOR DEALING WITH SYMPHYSIS PUBIS DYSFUNCTION PAIN

- Pelvic floor exercises can help tone muscles and prevent excessive movement of the pubis symphysis during pregnancy. Ideally begin before you become pregnant.

- Take up Pilates or Tai Chi before you become pregnant; both will strengthen your core muscles. This may not prevent pelvic pain during your pregnancy, but it will help speed the recovery process afterwards.

- Move little and often. You may not feel the effects of what you are doing until later in the day or after you have gone to bed.

- Rest regularly by sitting on a gym ball or by getting down on your hands and knees. This takes the weight of your baby off your pelvis and holds it in a stable position.

- Try not to do any heavy lifting or pushing. Supermarket trolleys can often make your pain worse, so shop online or shop little and often.

- Wear a pelvic support belt (available online, or your local pharmacy will be able to order one for you).

Pelvic pain in pregnancy responds very favourably to acupuncture treatment. Self-help or self-acupressure beyond what is discussed above is in most cases not possible due to the complex nature of this syndrome:

> Acupuncture, as an adjunct to standard treatment, was superior to standard treatment alone and physiotherapy in relieving mixed pelvic/back pain. Women with well-defined pelvic pain had greater relief of pain with a combination of acupuncture and standard treatment, compared to standard treatment alone or stabilizing exercises and standard treatment. (Ee *et al.* 2008)

Usually, the pelvic joint regains its stability gradually after your baby is born. The ligaments in the pelvic area become firmer once your body stops producing the hormone relaxin. As a result, the painful symptoms of SPD begin to subside slowly, eventually going away entirely.

BENEFITS OF ACUPUNCTURE

Acupuncture is superior to physiotherapy in the treatment of lower back pain and symphysis pubis pain

In the study by Elden *et al.* (2005), a total of 386 pregnant women were studied with the objective to compare the efficacy of standard treatment for pelvic pain (e.g. a pelvic belt, patient education and home exercises for the abdominal and gluteal muscles) with standard treatment plus acupuncture or standard treatment plus physiotherapy stabilising exercises (for the deep lumbar pelvic muscles).

The study time frame consisted of one week, which was used to establish a baseline, followed by six weeks of treatment. The acupuncture treatment was given twice a week and the stabilising exercise sessions one hour per week (with patients then doing these exercises several times a day on a daily basis).

The study concluded that acupuncture was superior to stabilising exercises in the management of pelvic girdle pain in pregnancy, with acupuncture the treatment of choice for patients with one-sided sacroiliac pain, one-sided sacroiliac pain combined with symphysis pubis pain, and bilateral sacroiliac pain.

Acupuncture decreases pain and improves women's ability to perform daily activities

Acupuncture was compared with non-penetrating sham acupuncture in women with pelvic girdle pain (PGP) during pregnancy by Elden *et al.* (2008). In a randomised double-blind controlled trial 115 pregnant women with PGP were randomly allocated to standard treatment plus acupuncture or to standard treatment plus non-penetrating sham acupuncture for eight weeks.

After treatment, median pain decreased in both groups (from 66 to 36 in the acupuncture group, and from 69 to 41 in the non-penetrating sham group), but there was no significant difference between groups.

Women in the acupuncture group were in regular work to a higher extent than women in the sham group, and the acupuncture group had superior ability to perform daily activities measured by the disability rating index.

Elden *et al.* conclude that acupuncture has no superior effect on pain relief, compared with sham acupuncture, but that it improved women's functional ability to perform daily activities.

Acupuncture is effective in treating pelvic or back pain in pregnancy

A systematic review of the effectiveness of acupuncture in treating pelvic and back pain in pregnancy has found evidence, although limited, which supports the use of acupuncture in treating these conditions. Two small trials on mixed pelvic and back pain and one large high-quality trial on pelvic pain met the inclusion criteria (see Ee *et al.* 2008).

Acupuncture relieves pelvic pain better than usual prenatal care

A systematic review using the Cochrane database has assessed the effects of interventions for preventing and treating back and pelvic pain in pregnancy (Pennick and Liddle 2007).

Pennick and Liddle searched the Cochrane database for randomised controlled trials of any treatment used to prevent or reduce the incidence or severity of back or pelvic pain in pregnancy. Eight studies (1305 participants from five countries) were included in the analysis.

Strengthening exercises, sitting pelvic tilt exercises and water gymnastics reduced pain intensity and back pain-related sick leave better than usual prenatal care alone. Both acupuncture and stabilising exercises relieved pelvic pain better than usual prenatal care, and acupuncture gave more relief from evening pain than exercises. One study found that acupuncture was more effective than physiotherapy in reducing the pain intensity scores of women with combined pelvic and back pain.

Sixty per cent of those who received acupuncture reported reduced pain compared with 14 per cent of those receiving usual care. No complications were associated with the use of acupuncture in pregnant women. Women who received usual prenatal care alone reported more use of analgesics, physical modalities and sacroiliac belts.

Acupuncture causes a decrease in pregnancy-related pelvic pain

Acupuncture has previously been shown to be more effective than either standard or specialised exercises in relieving pelvic pain in pregnancy (Elden et al. 2005). Now a new study has compared subcutaneous needling without further stimulation and deep needling for the same problem (see Lund et al. 2006).

Both groups experienced significant improvements in levels of pain intensity at rest and in daily activities as well as in rated emotional reaction and loss of energy, but there was no difference between the two different methods of acupuncture.

Acupuncture and the treatment of pelvic pain in pregnancy

In a Swedish study by Kvorning *et al.* (2004), 72 pregnant women (24–37 weeks) suffering pelvic or lower back pain were randomly assigned to an acupuncture group or a control group.

Traditional acupuncture points and Ah shi points were needled in individualised treatments, once or twice a week, until the disappearance of symptoms or delivery in the acupuncture group. Treatment was given for at least three weeks, twice weekly for the first two weeks, then once a week. The control group received no treatment.

During the study period the pain decreased in 60 per cent of patients in the acupuncture group compared to 14 per cent of the controls, dropping to 43 and 9 per cent respectively at the end of the study.

Acupuncture may be more effective than physiotherapy for pregnancy-related low-back and pelvic pain

Sixty pregnant women with low-back and pelvic pain were randomised to receive ten treatments of either acupuncture (30-minute sessions, given within one month) or physiotherapy (50-minute sessions of counselling and physical therapies, given within 6 to 8 weeks) (see Wedenberg, Moen and Norling 2000).

Significant improvements were noted in pain and in the ability to perform daily activities in the acupuncture group. The physiotherapy group had less pain relief but symptoms did not become worse (as they often do in pregnancy).

While the physiotherapy group had a high drop-out rate, which weakened the analysis, the researchers conclude that acupuncture is 'promising enough to warrant further studies'.

REFERENCES AND FURTHER READING

Ee, C. C., Manheimer, E., Pirotta, M. V. and White, A. R. (2008) 'Acupuncture for pelvic and back pain in pregnancy: A systematic review.' *American Journal of Obstetrics & Gynecology 198*, 3, 254–259.

Elden, H., Fagevik-Olsen, M., Ostgaard, H.-C., Stener-Victorin, E. and Hagberg, H. (2008) 'Acupuncture as an adjunct to standard treatment for pelvic girdle pain in pregnant women: Randomised double-blinded controlled trial comparing acupuncture with non-penetrating sham acupuncture.' *BJOG: An International Journal of Obstetrics & Gynaecology 115*, 13, 1655–1668.

Elden, H., Ladfors, L., Fagevik-Olsen, M., Ostgaard, H.-C. and Hagberg, H. (2005) 'Effects of acupuncture and stabilising exercises as adjunct to standard treatment in pregnant women with pelvic girdle pain: Randomised single-blind controlled trial.' *BMJ 330*, 7494, 761.

Kvorning, N., Holmberg, C., Grennert, L., Aberg, A. and Akeson, J. (2004) 'Acupuncture relieves pelvic and low-back pain in late pregnancy.' *Acta Obstetricia et Gynecologica Scandinavica 83*, 3, 246–250.

Lund, I., Lundeberg, T., Lönnberg, L. and Svensson, E. (2006) 'Decrease of pregnant women's pelvic pain after acupuncture: A randomized controlled single-blind study.' *Acta Obstetricia et Gynecologica Scandinavica 85*, 1, 12–19.

Pennick, V. and Liddle, S. D. (2007) 'Interventions for preventing and treating pelvic and back pain in pregnancy.' *Cochrane Database of Systematic Reviews 1*, 8, CD001139.

Wedenberg, K., Moen, B. and Norling, Å. (2000) 'A prospective randomized study comparing acupuncture with physiotherapy for low-back and pelvic pain in pregnancy.' *Acta Obstetricia et Gynecologica Scandinavica 79*, 331–335.

Chapter 11

POLYCYSTIC OVARIAN SYNDROME

POLYCYSTIC OVARIAN SYNDROME IN BIOMEDICINE

Polycystic ovarian syndrome (PCOS) affects up to 12 per cent of women of reproductive age, and up to 75 per cent of women suffering from infertility due to poor ovarian function (anovulation). The name 'polycystic ovarian syndrome' can be slightly misleading as it is systemic and has many manifestations. Because there is such a wide range of symptoms associated with PCOS, getting a diagnosis can be a time-consuming and frustrating experience.

Even though PCOS is a comparatively new syndrome (first documented in 1935), until 2003 there was no one specific diagnostic test or one presenting symptom that would confirm a clinical diagnosis. In 2003 standardised diagnostic criteria (the Rotterdam criteria) for diagnosing PCOS were developed.

According to the Rotterdam criteria, PCOS can be diagnosed if any two out of three criteria are met, in the absence of other entities that might cause these findings:

- Oligoovulation (infrequent or irregular ovulation) and/or anovulation (absence of ovulation)

- Excess androgen (male hormone) activity

- Polycystic ovaries.

WHAT CAUSES POLYCYSTIC OVARIAN SYNDROME?

The cause of PCOS is unknown, but most researchers think that several factors, including genetics, may have a role to play. It is generally agreed, however, that PCOS is an endocrine (hormonal) disorder. It is easy to see how easily a hormonal imbalance can wreak havoc in your body if you look at the extremely tight tolerances that your endocrine system works to. Hormones are measured in pictograms per millilitre of blood (pg/ml). That's one *trillionth* of a gram per millilitre. The difference between baseline oestrogen of 50 pg/ml and the ovulatory peak of 250 pg/ml is 200 trillionths of a gram, or 0.0000002 milligrams.

Family history

Immediate female relatives (i.e. daughters or sisters) of women with PCOS have up to a 50 per cent chance of having PCOS. No clear genetic contributor to PCOS is currently identified, and the link is likely to be complex and involve multiple genes.

Insulin resistance

Insulin is a hormone that controls the body's ability to metabolise (break down and then use or store for later) sugars. Many women with PCOS have an impaired ability to metabolise glucose, leading to insulin resistance and an increased production of androgens (male hormones). High androgen levels (hyperandrogenism) can lead to the development and maintenance of male characteristics and interfere with the normal production of female hormones such as oestrogen and progesterone. Research shows that approximately three-quarters of patients with PCOS have evidence of hyperandrogenism.

Poor sleep patterns

Poor sleep patterns have an extremely disruptive effect on hormonal function. When you don't get adequate sleep, one of the first things to be affected is your adrenal glands; these are responsible for proper steroid hormone (androgen) synthesis.

Poor liver and bowel function

Essential nutrients that support nervous, circulatory and endocrine function all need to be absorbed by the small intestine.

The liver acts as a filter, screening out degraded hormones as well as other waste products that are circulating in the blood. It then passes these waste products to the large intestine so that they can be removed from the body. Any backlog or inflammation in the gut affects levels of B vitamins essential for nervous system function, as well as trace minerals crucial for glandular function.

COMMON SYMPTOMS

Many women with PCOS will experience some of the following symptoms; however, you do not have to experience these symptoms to have PCOS, as some women have no symptoms at all:

- Irregular or totally absent periods (amenorrhoea). An irregular menstrual cycle is defined as either:

  - eight or less menstrual cycles per year

  - menstrual cycles longer than 35 days.

- Acne: The higher level of androgens (male hormones) present with PCOS can increase the size of the oil production glands in the skin, leading to acne.

- Hair loss (androgenic alopecia): A high level of androgens (male hormones) can cause male-pattern-type baldness, a receding frontal hair line and thinning on the top of the scalp.

- Excessive facial and body hair (hirsutism): This excess hair growth on the face and body is due to high levels of androgens stimulating the hair follicles. This excess hair is thicker and darker. The hair typically grows in areas where it is more usual for men to grow hair such as the chin, upper lip, around the nipples, lower abdomen, chest and thighs. Women with PCOS from ethnic groups prone to darker body hair, for example from the Mediterranean region, often find they are more severely affected by hirsutism.

- A darkening and thickening of areas of the skin (acanthosis nigricans): This may be especially noticeable in areas where there are skin folds, for example in the arm pit or groin.

- Breast disorders: A study conducted at the University of Rome (D'Amelio *et al.* 2001) found an association between PCOS and fibrocystic breast disease, based on ultrasounds of the pelvis and breasts. According to the ultrasound findings, only 6.8 per cent of women with normal ovaries had breast pathology, whereas 57 per cent of those with polycystic-appearing ovaries had breast pathology and 91 per cent of those with polycystic ovary syndrome also had breast pathology. (None of the women were using oral contraceptives.)

- Impaired glucose metabolism, glucose intolerance, insulin resistance: Patients with PCOS present a higher risk for abnormalities of glucose metabolism such as type 2 diabetes and metabolic syndrome (both PCOS and metabolic syndrome are associated with insulin resistance).

- Enlarged ovaries covered with cysts: It is from these cysts that the disorder gets its name. The current most cited ultrasonograpy criteria for PCOS is more than 10 cysts measuring 2–8 mm (0.08–0.3 inches) around or within a dense core of stroma.

- Fertility: High levels of androgens and high insulin levels can affect the menstrual cycle and prevent ovulation (the release of a mature egg from the ovaries). This can make it more difficult for women with PCOS to conceive naturally, and some women can also have a greater risk of miscarriage. However, this does not mean that all women with PCOS are infertile.

- Increased risk of diabetes in pregnancy (gestational diabetes): A condition of high glucose levels during pregnancy.

- Psychological effects: Depression and anxiety are common symptoms of PCOS. Approximately 29 per cent of women with PCOS have depression compared to around 7 per cent of women in the general population, and 57 per cent of women with PCOS will have anxiety compared to 18 per cent of women in the general population.

There may be some link to hormones, but more research is needed before this is fully understood.

HOW POLYCYSTIC OVARIAN SYNDROME AFFECTS FERTILITY

PCOS is a very complex condition marked by a complex web of multiple hormone imbalances. Hormones including insulin, androgens, oestrogen, progesterone, luteinising hormone (LH), follicle-stimulating hormone (FSH), adrenal hormones, thyroid hormones and prolactin, among others, all have to interact in a very precise way in order for pregnancy to occur. This interaction allows the formation and maturation of follicles (the structure within the ovary that produces the egg). The main difference between polycystic and normal ovaries is that although the polycystic ovaries contain many small follicles (antral follicles) with eggs in them, the follicles do not develop and mature properly, so there is no ovulation.

POLYCYSTIC OVARIAN SYNDROME IN CHINESE MEDICINE

In general, women with PCOS display a relative deficiency of Kidney Yin (oestrogen) and a relative excess of Kidney Yang (testosterone). It is this basic imbalance that accounts for the majority of the symptoms of PCOS.

If the movement of fluids are impaired due to the above Kidney imbalances, this can lead to secondary patterns marked by the presence of Dampness or Phlegm.

Cysts are usually fluid-filled sacs that tend to be more Damp Phlegm, but can sometimes be chocolate cysts or blood-filled cysts that are associated with Blood stasis.

Amenorrhoea (no period) and failure to shed the uterine lining each month can lead to Qi and Blood stagnation.

DIETARY CONSIDERATIONS

As PCOS is strongly influenced by insulin levels and glucose metabolism, diet and lifestyle modifications can have a significant impact on balancing hormones and regulating blood sugar levels and PCOS.

- Eat foods low on the glycaemic index such as vegetables and whole grains. Try to avoid refined carbohydrates that include sugar (hidden in most processed foods), white flour and whole wheat flour, and products made from them (pasta, breads, etc.). These foods will cause insulin levels to spike rapidly and lead to an increased production of androgens (male hormones).

- Consume complex carbohydrates such as whole grain cereals, quinoa, brown rice or millet, rather than simple carbohydrates such as white rice. Complex carbohydrates break down at a gradual rate and do not spike blood sugar levels.

- Keep your blood sugar stable by eating regularly – ideally every three to five hours.

- Eat at least two portions of leafy greens a day (kale, broccoli, cabbage, etc.). Leafy greens contain indole-3-carbinol, which helps to regulate liver function, which is key in glucose and hormone metabolism.

- If you eat red meat make sure it comes from grass-fed animals. When meat has been grain fed it changes the fats from healthy omega-3 fats to omega-6 fats that are unhealthy in excess.

- Eat berries rather than fruit – these are lower on the glycaemic index (and tend to be higher in antioxidants).

- Ensure you have an adequate fibre intake (30 g (1 oz)/day), by eating lots of fresh vegetables and whole grains.

Foods to avoid

If you can eliminate these foods for a week, and you notice a flatter stomach, more energy and a more regular bowel movement, you may be intolerant to one or more of them. Add them back in one by one and you'll discover the culprit(s). Ideally, however, totally eliminate refined carbohydrates from your diet (although you can have a cheat meal on special occasions):

- Refined sugars (white and brown sugars, fructose, sucrose, corn syrup) and simple sugars (maple syrup, honey, etc.).

- Refined carbohydrates (white bread, pasta, potatoes, white rice, processed breakfast cereals, rice cakes, popcorn, or any starchy, low-fibre food).

- Artificial sweeteners (which are shown to affect the insulin levels the same way as sugar).

- Milk and dairy products. Try substituting unsweetened almond milk as an alternative to cow's milk. Green vegetables will more than meet your calcium requirements.

VITAMIN AND MINERAL SUPPLEMENTS

Vitamin B complex: Can help to restore normal liver function in insulin balancing.

Chlorophyll: Reduces symptoms of hypoglycaemia without raising blood glucose level. Remember that it is very cold in nature, so take it with some chai tea to counteract this.

Chromium: Essential in proper carbohydrate metabolism. Insufficiency may result in insulin resistance.

Cinnamon: A rich source of antioxidants that can help improve blood glucose control.

Fennel: Metformin (mefenamic acid) is used to improve insulin sensitivity and lower insulin levels, which directly affects anovulation and hyperandrogenism. Fennel acts in a similar way to mefenamic acid, but without the side effects.

Magnesium: Clinical research has established a connection between magnesium deficiency and insulin resistance.

Omega-3 fatty acids: Found to reduce testosterone levels in women with PCOS.

Zinc: Needed for correct hormone balance and thyroid function.

THERAPEUTIC RECIPES

For a complete listing of the energetic qualities and uses in Chinese medicine of most common foods, see Appendix A.

The focus of the majority of the recipes below is draining Dampness (oedema). One of the major complications of PCOS is the accumulated Dampness preventing normal interaction between the various aspects of the reproductive system. The fluid build-up means that Qi cannot move in a normal fashion, and this leads to stagnation (cysts).

Breakfast

Porridge made with water and sprinkled with cinnamon. Porridge is warming in nature; it improves digestive function and Blood circulation. Cinnamon improves Blood circulation in the smaller vessels such as those in the fingers, toes or around the reproductive organs.

Walnuts and/or cashews in natural yoghurt. Although yoghurt is considered cold in nature, both walnuts and cashews are warming. It is important to choose yoghurt with no added sugar and live bacteria.

Lunch

Salad: Many salad vegetables are cold in nature (this can slow down digestive function and impair the movement of Qi and Blood), but the addition of onions, garlic, ginger, chilli or peppers can mediate the cooling action of the vegetables.

Try some of the following combinations:

Carrot, apple and ginger

Carrot and radish

Duck, watercress and orange

Guacamole

Mixed beans with chilli

Prawns with bean sprouts

Dinner

RED BEAN SOUP

Ingredients

- 200 g (8 oz) adzuki beans
- 1½ litres (6 cups) water
- 1 large piece of fresh orange peel
- 1 cm (½ inch) fresh root ginger, grated or finely chopped

Method

1. Soak the adzuki beans in water overnight to soften. (While the beans won't have completely softened, they will have expanded considerably.) Drain.

2. Bring the water to a boil in a pan. (The soup can be thicker or thinner as desired; just add more boiling water at the end of cooking to thin it a bit if required.)

3. Turn the heat down, add the adzuki beans and simmer, partially covered, for 1–1½ hours, until the beans are softened to the point where they are just beginning to break apart.

4. Add the orange peel and ginger. Serve.

Therapeutic qualities

Adzuki beans: Drain Dampness (reduce oedema).

Orange peel: Supports proper digestive function and drains Dampness.

Ginger: Moves Qi and reinforces the Damp-draining effects of the adzuki beans and orange peel.

PORK AND MUNG BEAN SOUP

Ingredients

- 450 g (1 lb) pork spare ribs, cut into 2.5 cm (1 inch) lengths
- 1 tsp Szechuan peppercorns
- 1½ litres (6 cups) water
- 100 g (3½ oz) mung beans, rinsed, soaked in warm water for 40 minutes and drained
- 1 cm (½ inch) fresh root ginger, grated or finely chopped
- 1 spring onion (scallion)
- 20 g (0.7 oz) seaweed, chopped into pieces
- sea salt

Method

1. Blanch the spare ribs with the peppercorns in boiling water for a few minutes. Remove and drain.

2. Heat a large saucepan with water over a high heat. Add the spare ribs, mung beans, ginger and spring onions, and bring to the boil.

3. Turn the heat down and cover the pan. Simmer for about 3 hours. Add the seaweed.

4. Simmer for 30 minutes more. Season and serve.

Therapeutic qualities

Pork ribs: Nourish Yin.

Szechuan peppercorns: Moves Qi; the warm nature of the pepper mediates the cooling nature of the pork, mung beans and seaweed.

Mung beans: Drain Dampness (oedema) and clear Heat (inflammation).

Ginger and spring onion: Move Qi and Blood; their warm aromatic nature allows them to dispel Dampness (oedema).

Seaweed: Nourishes Yin while it drains Dampness (oedema).

PINEAPPLE TOFU

Ingredients

- 2 tbsp soy sauce
- 100 ml (4 fl oz) pineapple juice
- 2 tbsp olive oil
- 1 clove garlic, grated or finely chopped
- 1.5 cm (0.6 inches) fresh root ginger, grated or finely chopped
- 150 g (5 oz) firm tofu, diced into cubes
- 50 g (2 oz) pineapple pieces
- 2 tsp cornflour (cornstarch)

Method

1. Whisk together the soy sauce and pineapple juice.

2. Using the olive oil, fry the garlic, ginger and tofu until the tofu is lightly browned. Reduce the heat and add the pineapple sauce and pineapple pieces, stirring well to combine. Heat for 2–3 minutes, then add the cornflour.

3. Heat for 1 more minute until the sauce thickens. Serve.

Therapeutic qualities

Pineapple: Clears Heat (inflammation) and produces Body Fluids.

Tofu: Clears Heat (inflammation) and produces Body Fluids.

Ginger: Moves Qi and Body Fluids; its warm nature mediates the cooling nature of the other ingredients.

Soy sauce: Clears Heat (inflammation).

BONE MARROW SOUP

Ingredients

- 500 g (1 lb) pork or chicken bones
- 1 tbsp goji berries
- 50 g (2 oz) pearl barley
- 1 stalk lemongrass
- 1 tbsp apple cider vinegar

Method

1. Add all the ingredients to a pot and bring to the boil.
2. Simmer for 1 hour.
3. Strain and serve.

Therapeutic qualities

Pork: Nourishes Yin and Blood.

Chicken: Blood and Qi tonic.

Goji berries: Support the pork in nourishing Yin.

Pearl barley: Drains Dampness (stagnated fluids).

Lemongrass: Its aromatic nature moves Qi and prevents the soup becoming too cloying (Damp forming).

Apple cider vinegar: Leaches nutrients from the bones as well as helps prevent the loss of minerals (which in most cases are Yin tonics).

 SPICY SPINACH

Ingredients

- 1 bunch spinach, washed and chopped
- 1 tsp wasabi paste
- 1 tbsp soy sauce
- 1 tbsp rice vinegar
- 1 tbsp sesame oil

Method

1. Pour boiling water over the spinach to wilt it and leave to cool.
2. Squeeze out the excess water, and place the spinach in a serving bowl.

3. Prepare the dressing by combining the wasabi paste, soy sauce, vinegar and sesame oil in a small bowl and stir well.

4. Toss the spinach in the dressing and serve.

Therapeutic qualities

Spinach: Qi and Blood tonic.

Wasabi: Moves Qi and Blood. Its warm nature mediates the cool nature of spinach.

Soy sauce: Clears Heat (inflammation).

Sesame oil: Tonifies Kidney Qi.

Rice vinegar: Acts as an astringent balancing the action of the other ingredients.

 ## SESAME DUCK SALAD

Ingredients

- five spice marinade (see below)
- 1 duck breast
- 100 g (3½ oz) noodles
- 1 tbsp olive oil
- handful of peas
- 1 carrot, grated
- 1 spring onion (scallion), finely sliced
- 1 tsp sesame seeds, toasted

FIVE SPICE MARINADE

- 1 tbsp sesame oil
- 1 tsp five spice powder
- 1 tsp brown sugar
- 1 tbsp rice wine vinegar
- 1 clove garlic, grated or finely chopped
- 1 tbsp soy sauce

Method

1. Make the marinade by mixing all the ingredients together in a bowl.

2. Slice the duck breast into bite-size pieces and allow to marinate in the mix for 30 minutes (or overnight is even better).

3. Cook the noodles in boiling, salted water until tender. Drain, rinse and set aside.

4. Add the olive oil to a wok or frying pan and stir-fry the duck breast until cooked.

5. Steam the peas and carrot until just tender.

6. Mix all the ingredients in a bowl and toss together. Garnish with the spring onion and sesame seeds. Serve.

Therapeutic qualities

Duck: Regulates the Triple Burner (San Jiao). This allows proper fluid metabolism.

Peas: Drain Dampness (oedema) by promoting diuresis.

Carrot: Nourishes Yin and Blood. While you drain Dampness it is important not to damage Body Fluids.

Five spice powder: Cinnamon moves Qi and Blood in the smaller vessels, cloves break Blood stasis, Szechuan peppercorns tonify Qi, fennel seeds envoy to the lower Jiao and star anise tonifies Qi.

Rice wine vinegar: Stops bleeding.

Soy sauce: Clears Heat (inflammation).

Sesame seeds and oil: Envoy to the pelvic region.

Spring onions: Regulate Qi and Blood circulation.

Brown sugar: Harmonises the digestive system.

Garlic: Moves Qi and Blood, and counteracts the damp-forming tendencies of the brown sugar.

 ## FRIED BEEF WITH CELERY

Ingredients

- 200 g (7 oz) beef (good quality, suitable for fast cooking)
- soy sauce
- 1 tbsp cornflour (cornstarch)
- 2 sticks celery
- 2 tbsp sesame oil

Method

1. Shred the beef and cover in a soy sauce and cornflour mix.

2. Slice the celery into bite-size pieces and boil until just tender.

3. Heat the sesame oil in a wok or frying pan and cook the beef to your liking. Add the celery and serve.

Therapeutic qualities

Beef: Qi and Blood tonic.

Celery: Clears Heat (inflammation) and drains Dampness (oedema) by promoting diuresis.

Sesame oil: Tonifies Kidney Qi.

Soy sauce: Clears Heat (inflammation).

ACUPRESSURE

How to apply pressure to the points

To press points, use something blunt. You can use finger pressure, but if you have to apply sustained pressure, you may find it uncomfortable. A chopstick (like the ones you get with a takeaway meal) is ideal for this purpose.

Ideally have someone do the treatment for you; that way you are not creating muscular tension while you try and reach points. You can also focus more on what sensations (or lack of them) result from pressing the point.

Don't press too hard; use enough pressure that you (or your partner) can feel something happening.

When you get to the point where something is happening, keep the pressure constant and hold for 30 seconds.

If you are not feeling any effects from pressing a point, you may not be pressing on the exact right spot. Try different spots around the location you first tried.

The points

There are any number of points that can be used, and in most cases points used in an acupuncture treatment are selected based on signs and symptoms presenting at that time. The points listed below are all useful in the treatment of PCOS, but for a more individualised treatment plan, talk to a licensed acupuncture practitioner.

STOMACH 40 (FENG LONG) ABUNDANT BULGE

Actions – Transforms Phlegm and Dampness.

Location – Eight finger breadths superior to the tip of the external malleolus lateral to Stomach 38 (Tiao Kou), approximately two finger breadths lateral to the anterior border of the tibia.

Location note – The point is half way up your shin (measure from the ankle crease) and two finger breadths out.

LIVER 4 (ZHONG FENG) MIDDLE SEAL

Actions – Spreads Liver Qi, regulates the lower Jiao and clears stagnant Heat.

Location – Anterior to the medial malleolus midway between Spleen 5 (Shang Qiu) and Stomach 41 (Jie Xi) in the depression on the medial side of the tendon of the tibialis anterior muscle.

Location note – Draw a line from the bottom edge of your ankle bone (inside one) straight across the crease. As you run your finger across this line there is a bump; this is the tibialis anterior tendon. The point is on the inside of the tendon on the line that you have drawn. A number of points on this line are good to drain Dampness.

LIVER 9 (YIN BAO) YIN BLADDER

Actions – Clears Liver Qi stagnation affecting the genital region and/or reproductive organs.

Location – Four finger breadths above the medial epicondyle of the femur between the vastus medialis and sartorius muscles.

Location note – The point is four finger breadths above the ankle bone (inside one) on the inside edge of your shin bone.

LIVER 13 (ZHANG MEN) CAMPHOR WOOD GATE

Actions – Harmonises the Liver and Spleen, regulates the middle and lower Jiao.

Location – On the lateral side of the abdomen, below the free end of the eleventh rib.

Location note – This rib is hard to find as it is very short. Start on the upper abdomen where you can feel the lower edge of the ribcage and follow it down.

KIDNEY 3 (TAI XI) GREAT RAVINE

Actions – Nourishes Kidney Yin and Yang, clears Empty Heat.

Location – In the depression between the tip of the medial malleolus (ankle bone, on the inside of the ankle) and the Achilles tendon. In many women there is a noticeable depression over the point.

KIDNEY 5 (SHUI QUAN) WATER SPRING

Actions – Regulates the Chong and Ren Mai and benefits menstruation.

Location – One finger breadth directly below Kidney 3 (Tai Xi), in the depression of the medial side of the tuberosity of the calcaneum.

Location note – Find Kidney 3 (Tai Xi) (above), and drop down one finger breadth.

GALL BLADDER 26 (DAI MAI) GIRDLING VESSEL

Actions – Regulates the Dai Mai (Belt Vessel) and drains Dampness, regulates menstruation and stops leucorrhoea.

Location – Directly below Liver 13 (Zhang Men) at the crossing point of a vertical line through the free end of the eleventh rib and a horizontal line drawn through the umbilicus.

Location note – Draw a line from the centre of your armpit straight down towards your hip, and another from your belly button across. The point is where the lines intersect.

ADJUNCT SELF-TREATMENTS

Ovarian massage

The ovaries lie approximately 10 cm (4 inches) down from the navel and 7 cm (3 inches) from the midline. Massage the area in a circular motion; apply as much pressure as you can without causing pain. Pressure can be applied with your finger tips in a circular kneading motion.

REFERENCES AND FURTHER READING

Atiomo, W. U., El-Mahdi, E. and Hardiman, P. (2003) 'Familial associations in women with polycystic ovary syndrome.' *Fertility and Sterility 80*, 143–145.

Botsis, D., Kassanos, D., Pyrgiotis, E. and Zourlas, P. A. (1995) 'Sonographic incidence of polycystic ovaries in gynecological population.' *Ultrasound in Obstetrics & Gynecology 6*, 182–185.

Clayton, R. N., Ogden, V., Hodgkinson, J. *et al.* (1992) 'How common are polycystic ovaries in normal women and what is their significance for the fertility of the population?' *Clinical Endocrinology 37*, 127–134.

Cole, P., Elwood, J. M. and Kaplan, S. D. (1978) 'Incidence rates and risk factors of benign breast neoplasms.' *American Journal of Epidemiology 108*, 112–120.

Cresswell, J. L., Barker, D. J., Osmond, C., Egger, P., Phillips, D. I. and Fraser, R. B. (1997) 'Fetal growth, length of gestation, and polycystic ovaries in adult life.' *The Lancet 350*, 1131–1135.

D'Amelio, R., Farris, M., Grande, S., Feraudo, E., Iuliano, A. and Zichella, L. (2001) 'Association between polycystic ovary and fibrocystic breast disease.' *Gynecologic and Obstetric Investigation 51*, 134–137.

Farquhar, C. M., Birdsall, M., Manning, P., Mitchell, J. M. and France, J. T. (1994) 'The prevalence of polycystic ovaries on ultrasound scanning in a population of randomly selected women.' *Australian and New Zealand Journal of Obstetrics & Gynaecology 34*, 1277–1279.

Fleming, N. T., Armstrong, B. K. and Sheiner, H. J. (1982) 'The comparative epidemiology of benign breast lumps and breast cancer in Western Australia.' *International Journal of Cancer 30*, 147–152.

Homberg, R. (2003) 'The management of infertility associated with polycystic ovary syndrome.' *Reproductive Biology and Endocrinology 1*, 109.

Jick, S. S., Walker, A. M. and Jick, H. (1986) 'Conjugated estrogens and fibrocystic breast disease.' *American Journal of Epidemiology 124*, 746–751.

Lyttleton, J. (2004) *Treatment of Infertility with Chinese Medicine.* Edinburgh: Churchill Livingstone.

Maciocia, G. (1998) *Obstetrics and Gynecology in Chinese Medicine.* Edinburgh: Churchill Livingstone.

Namavar Jahromi, B., Tartifizadeh, A. and Khabnadideh, S. (2003) 'Comparison of fennel and mefenamic acid for the treatment of primary dysmenorrhea.' *International Journal of Gynaecology and Obstetrics 80*, 2, 153–157.

Ory, H., Cole, P., MacMahon, B. and Hoover, R. (1976) 'Oral contraceptives and reduced risk of benign breast diseases.' *New England Journal of Medicine 294*, 419.

Pierpoint, T., McKeigue, P. M., Isaacs, A. J., Wild, S. H. and Jacobs, H. S. (1998) 'Mortality of women with polycystic ovary syndrome at long-term follow-up.' *Journal of Clinical Epidemiology 51*, 581–586.

Polson, D. W., Adams, J., Wadsworth, J. and Franks, S. (1988) 'Polycystic ovaries – A common finding in normal women.' *The Lancet 1*, 870–872.

Sheehan, M. T. (2003) 'Polycystic ovarian syndrome: Diagnosis and management.' *Chinese Medicine & Research 1*, 13–27.

Soran, A., Talbott, E. O., Zborowski, J. V. and Wilson, J. W. (2005) 'The prevalence of benign breast disease in women with polycystic ovary syndrome: A review of a 12-year follow-up.' *The International Journal of Clinical Practice 59*, 7, 795–797.

Talbott, E., Guzick, D., Clerici, A. *et al.* (1995) 'Coronary heart disease risk factors in women with polycystic ovary syndrome.' *Arteriosclerosis, Thrombosis, and Vascular Biology 7*, 821–827.

Tayob, Y., Robinson, G., Adams, J. *et al.* (1990) 'Ultrasound appearance of the ovaries during the pill-free interval.' *British Journal of Family Planning 16*, 94–96.

Wild, S., Pierpoint, T., Jacobs, H. and McKeigue, P. (2000) 'Long-term consequences of polycystic ovary syndrome: Results of a 31 year follow-up study.' *Human Fertility (Cambridge) 3*, 101–105.

Chapter 12

PREMENSTRUAL SYNDROME

Premenstrual syndrome (PMS) is a collection of emotional symptoms, with or without physical symptoms, related to a woman's menstrual cycle. Most women of reproductive age experience altered physical and/or mental states around ovulation or in the lead up to a period at some time in their lives; however, up to 10 per cent of women have symptoms that severely disrupt their lives.

These symptoms are usually termed 'premenstrual syndrome'. The more the scientific community learns about PMS, the more a hormonal imbalance is thought to be the primary culprit. The exact symptoms and their intensity vary significantly from woman to woman, and even somewhat from cycle to cycle. Most women with PMS experience only a few of the possible symptoms, in a relatively predictable pattern.

DIAGNOSIS OF PREMENSTRUAL SYNDROME

There is no laboratory test or unique physical findings to verify the diagnosis, and more than 200 different symptoms have been associated with PMS, but the criteria set out by Steiner *et al.* (2011) are often used to make a definitive diagnosis.

Diagnosis of PMS is based on the presence of at least five symptoms, including one of four core symptoms, from a list of 17 physical and psychological core symptoms.

The 17 symptoms are:

- Depression

- Feeling hopeless or guilty

- Anxiety/tension

- Mood swings

- Irritability/persistent anger

- Decreased interest in life generally

- Poor concentration

- Fatigue

- Food craving or increased appetite

- Sleep disturbance

- Feeling out of control or overwhelmed

- Poor coordination

- Headache

- Muscle aches

- Swelling/bloating/weight gain

- Abdominal cramping

- Breast tenderness.

RISK FACTORS FOR PREMENSTRUAL SYNDROME

Most researchers have also put forth the theory that PMS is caused primarily by cultural factors, as it is much more common in the Western world.

Other factors thought to play a role are:

- High caffeine intake: Caffeine strips nutrients (especially minerals) from the body. Low nutrient levels can lead to hormonal imbalances that can cause or aggravate the symptoms of PMS.

- Dietary factors: Low levels of certain vitamins and minerals, particularly vitamins B6, D and E, magnesium, manganese and zinc.

- Stress: Everyone has a different view of stress. 'Being stressed out' is a very individual emotional state. At mid and end cycle, when hormones are in a state of flux, stress can cause these hormonal shifts to be especially noticeable.

- Increasing age: Hormone balances naturally alter as women age, and the symptoms of PMS may become worse as a result of these altered hormonal balances. In some cases premenstrual-type symptoms only begin in perimenopause.

- Family history: There may be a genetic aspect to the probability of having PMS.

VITAMIN AND MINERAL SUPPLEMENTS

Vitamin B6: A number of studies have shown the effectiveness of vitamin B6 on PMS. It plays a vital part in synthesising neurotransmitters (chemicals that control your mood and behaviour).

Vitamin E: Shown to be helpful for the breast symptoms associated with PMS and also mood swings and irritability.

Calcium: The most abundant, essential mineral in the body (approximately 2 per cent), and critical for many metabolic functions, such as the development and maintenance of teeth and bones, transmission of nerve impulses, control of the heartbeat and blood pressure, muscle relaxation and contraction and enzyme activation. Fluctuating oestrogen levels during the menstrual cycle may lead to a calcium imbalance (oestrogen regulates calcium metabolism). Calcium depletion may interact with oestrogen and progesterone after ovulation, giving rise to both hormonal imbalances and muscular aches.

Chromium: Needed for the metabolism and maintenance of proper blood sugar levels. Many of the symptoms of PMS can be caused or aggravated by blood sugar imbalances.

Magnesium: Nature's tranquilliser, and can easily treat symptoms such as anxiety, tension, irritability or depression, Taking magnesium daily starting two weeks before a period may improve the symptoms of PMS. Look for magnesium citrate, which is easier to absorb than magnesium oxide (taking magnesium with vitamin B6 will increase magnesium absorption).

Omega-3 fatty acids: It is now estimated that we are getting ten times more omega-6 fats from our diet than omega-3, and over the last century there has been an 80 per cent decrease in the consumption of these omega-3 fatty acids. When you eat omega-3 fats they are converted to substances that have an anti-inflammatory effect on the body, while omega-6 can promote inflammation. A considerable portion of the symptoms associated with PMS can be attributed to low-grade inflammation and/or hormonal imbalances. Supplementing with high-grade cold-pressed fish oils should bring about a significant reduction in symptoms.

A note about evening primrose oil: Evening primrose oil can contain high levels of inflammatory omega-6 fats. I have seen cases where symptoms of PMS have become worse as a result of taking excessive amounts of evening primrose oil. As a general rule, take supplements containing omega-3 fats rather than omega-6 as you will most likely have enough omega-6 in your system as a result of eating a standard Western diet.

DIETARY THERAPY

Foods containing natural plant sterols can be helpful. They are thought to block the oestrogen receptors, so in turn, excess oestrogen in the body cannot lock in to these receptors. These include:

- Peas, beans and pulses
- Garlic
- Apples
- Parsley

- Fennel

- Brassicas: cabbage, cauliflower, etc. Vegetables from the cabbage family in particular can increase the rate at which the liver changes oestrogen into a water-soluble form that is easily excreted

- Celery, carrots

- Rhubarb

- Sage.

Reduce or totally avoid:

- Caffeine: Limit beverages containing caffeine to one a day. If you suffer from lumpy or painful breasts, cut out caffeine completely.

- Reduce your alcohol intake: Restricting alcohol allows your liver to function more effectively. The liver is responsible for clearing excess hormones (which cause hormonal imbalance) from the bloodstream. Alcohol consumption contributes to blood sugar imbalance, which is implicated in PMS and other symptoms of hormonal imbalance.

As always with food sensitivities, cut out the offending foods for a month, and then reintroduce them slowly, one at a time. See how you react or not, and act accordingly.

PREMENSTRUAL SYNDROME IN CHINESE MEDICINE
In the Ming Dynasty (1368–1644 AD) Dan-Xi advised that to diagnose cases of feverish sensation in women's diseases one should ascertain whether it occurred during menstruation or at other times as well.

In Ye Tianshi's gynaecological records (also Ming Dynasty), premenstrual symptoms such as oedema, feverish sensation, pain in the hypochondrium, diarrhoea, body aches, abdominal cramps and reduced appetite were recorded.

According to Chinese medical theory, PMS is mostly indicative of a disharmony in the Liver. The main job the Liver is expected to do is to maintain the free flow of Qi and Blood. If the proper circulation of Qi is compromised, it results in symptoms that are recognisable as PMS.

The following common symptoms are likely to be caused by Qi stagnation:

- Mood swings

- Undirected anger

- Abdominal bloating

- Breast distension/lumps that appear around ovulation or periods

- Dull, aching abdominal or pelvic pain around ovulation (Mittelschmerz).

Caffeine is a popular self-treatment for breaking up Qi stagnation. Caffeine does move Qi, and break stagnation; however, after the caffeine hit wears off, the stagnation will return with greater intensity.

DIETARY TREATMENT IN CHINESE MEDICINE

- Eat little and often: Don't put the digestive system under pressure or Qi stagnations can result.

- Eat main meals earlier in the day: Early in the day (before 5pm) more Qi is available for digestion and Qi is active. There is less likelihood of stagnation.

- Small quantities (half a teaspoon) of spirit alcohol can be therapeutic as it moves stagnant Qi.

- Limit coffee to one cup a day, ideally first thing in the morning. Caffeine can be used to power up the digestive system for the coming day, as well as moving Qi that may be a bit sluggish after the relative inactivity of the night.

- Incorporate mildly dispersive, pungent flavours into your diet. These include onions, garlic, watercress, turmeric, basil, mint, peppermint, horseradish, pepper, cardamom, cumin, fennel, dill and ginger.

- Small quantities of sour flavours can be therapeutic, such as citrus fruits, vinegar and pickles.

- Eat plenty of fresh vegetables. Ideally green vegetables will make up a large percentage of your diet.

- Eat small amounts of high-quality protein and fish.

THERAPEUTIC RECIPES

For a complete listing of the energetic qualities and uses in Chinese medicine of most common foods, see Appendix A.

A large proportion of the symptoms of PMS can be attributed to Qi stagnation, and these symptoms are very commonly the cause of women attending clinic. The recipes listed below are all effective at moving stagnant Qi and should thus prevent or relieve the symptoms of PMS in the majority of cases. Ideally don't wait until you have symptoms; adjust your diet and begin to work on the points listed below around ovulation.

Breakfast

Porridge made with water and sprinkled with flaxseeds. Porridge is warming in nature; it improves digestive function and Blood circulation. Flaxseeds nourish Yin; they soften what is stuck and rigid.

Walnuts and/or cashews in natural yoghurt. Although yoghurt is considered cold in nature, both walnuts and cashews are warming. It is important to choose yoghurt with no added sugar and live bacteria.

Lunch

Salad: Many salad vegetables are cold in nature (this can slow down digestive function and impair the movement of Qi and Blood), but the addition of onions, garlic, ginger, chilli or peppers can mediate the cooling action of the vegetables.

Try some of the following combinations:

Carrot, apple and ginger

Carrot and radish

Duck, watercress and orange

Mixed beans with chilli

Guacamole

Prawns with bean sprouts

Dinner

 ### FENNEL AND TANGERINE SALAD

Ingredients

- 1 fennel bulb, finely sliced
- 1 small red onion, finely sliced
- 4 tangerines, peeled and separated into segments
- 1 pomegranate, seeds
- small bunch of parsley, finely chopped
- 1 lemon, juice
- ½ tbsp olive oil
- salt and pepper (optional)

Method

1. Mix all the ingredients together in a bowl.
2. Season and serve.

Therapeutic qualities

Fennel: Regulates the movement of Qi, especially in the pelvic region.

Onion: Moves Qi and aromaticity, dispels Dampness (oedema).

Parsley: Regulates Qi flow.

Tangerine: Its cool nature clears Heat.

Pomegranate: Clears Empty Heat (heat built up as a result of stagnation).

Lemon: Clears Empty Heat (heat built up as a result of stagnation).

SALMON AND GINGER FISHCAKES

Ingredients

- 140 g (5 oz) salmon fillet, finely chopped
- 2 tsp fresh root ginger, grated or finely chopped
- zest of 1 small lime
- 3 spring onions (scallions), finely sliced
- black pepper and sea salt
- 1 tsp sesame oil

Method

1. Mix the salmon in a bowl with the ginger, lime zest and spring onions, and season.

2. After chilling the mixture, form into patties.

3. Heat the oil in a frying pan and cook the patties for 3–4 minutes each side until golden and cooked through. Serve.

Therapeutic qualities

Salmon: Nourishes Yin; its cool nature clears Heat.

Sesame oil and ginger: Are warm in nature and balance the cold qualities of the salmon.

Spring onions and lime zest: Move Qi and prevent stagnation. Their warm nature reinforces the action of the sesame and ginger.

RED PRAWN CURRY

Ingredients

- curry paste, to taste (see below)
- 1 tbsp groundnut oil
- 100 ml (4 fl oz) coconut milk
- 5 cloves
- 1 onion, finely chopped
- 100 ml (4 fl oz) chicken stock
- 1 tsp peppercorns
- 1 tbsp fish sauce
- 1 tsp brown sugar
- 50 g (2 oz) bamboo shoots, chopped
- 100 g (3½ oz) raw tiger prawns
- red chilli, finely sliced

CURRY PASTE

- 1 stalk lemongrass, roughly chopped
- 1 small shallot, grated
- 1 clove garlic, grated or finely chopped
- 2 tsp galangal (or ginger), grated or finely chopped
- 3 tsp coriander seeds
- 1 lime leaf, shredded
- 1 tsp ground cumin
- 1 tbsp groundnut oil
- sea salt

Method

1. For the curry paste, blend all the ingredients into a smooth paste.

2. Heat the oil in a large frying pan. Add the curry paste and cook for 30 seconds to allow the aromas and flavours to release.

3. Add the coconut milk, cloves and onion, and cook for 3 minutes before adding the stock, peppercorns, fish sauce, brown sugar and bamboo shoots. Bring to the boil, turn down to a simmer and continue to cook for approximately 10 minutes. Add the tiger prawns and cook for a further 5 minutes.

4. Serve garnished with chilli.

Therapeutic qualities

Cloves, lemongrass, shallots, galangal, lime leaf, chilli and onion: All move Qi. Their warm nature mediates the cooling qualities of the bamboo shoots.

Coriander: Clears Empty Heat (a build-up of heat resulting from lack of Qi movement).

Cumin: Regulates the movement of Qi.

Prawns and brown sugar: Warm in nature, they tonify Qi while harmonising the digestive system.

Coconut milk: Nourishes Yin and moves Qi.

PORK AND SEAFOOD STEW

Ingredients (for 2 portions)

- 200 g (7 oz) pork belly, cut into bite-size pieces
- 1 clove garlic, grated or finely chopped
- 1 onion, finely chopped
- 1 red pepper (bell pepper), sliced
- 1 bulb fennel, sliced
- 1 tbsp olive oil
- 2 tsp cumin seeds
- pinch of saffron
- 2 tsp smoked paprika
- 2 tsp ground turmeric
- 2 tomatoes, chopped
- 1 tbsp tomato puree
- 1 l (35 fl oz) fish stock
- 1 lemon
- 50 g (2 oz) mussels
- 4 raw king prawns
- 1 squid, cleaned (ask your fishmonger to do this) and cut into bite-size pieces

Method

1. Mix the pork, garlic, onion, pepper and fennel in a pan and add olive oil.

2. Fry over a medium heat for a couple of minutes and then add the cumin seeds, saffron, paprika and turmeric.

3. Cook for 5 minutes and then add the tomatoes and tomato puree. Cook for a further 5 minutes, allowing the tomatoes to break down.

4. Add the stock, season and simmer for around 10 minutes.

5. Zest the lemon into the stew and add the juice.

6. Wash the mussels. Peel and de-vein the prawns. Add the shellfish to the pan and cook for 5 minutes. Serve.

Therapeutic qualities

Prawns and mussels: Qi tonics.

Pork: Yin and Blood tonic.

Squid: Liver Blood tonic.

Onion, garlic, lemon zest, turmeric, saffron and red pepper: Move Qi and prevent stagnation.

Tomatoes: Clear Heat and produce Body Fluids.

Fennel and cumin seeds: Regulate Qi flow.

Paprika: Harmonises the digestive system.

Lemon juice: Its cool nature prevents the shellfish and spices overheating the dish.

SPICY BAKED CHICKEN

Ingredients

- 3 tbsp sesame oil
- 4 chicken thighs, on the bone
- 1 onion, chopped
- 2 tsp ground white pepper
- 2 tsp cinnamon
- 4 cardamom pods, lightly crushed
- 1 tbsp parsley, finely chopped
- 4 tbsp curry paste (see above)

Method

1. Heat the oven to 190°C/Gas Mark 5/375°F.

2. Heat 1 tbsp of the oil in a large casserole dish with a lid. Add the chicken and cook until golden all over, then remove the chicken from the dish.

3. Fry the onion and spices in the remaining oil, until the onion is soft and golden. Then return the chicken to the dish.

4. Mix the parsley and curry paste together, and spoon over the chicken. Be sure that the chicken is coated in the spice mix (add a little more oil if you need to).

5. Put the lid on the dish and cook in a medium oven for 30 minutes, or until the meat falls easily off the bone.

Therapeutic qualities

Chicken and sesame oil: Qi tonics.

Onion, pepper, cinnamon and cardamom: Move Qi and prevent stagnation.

Parsley: Regulates the flow of Qi.

CHICKEN RENDANG

Ingredients

- 4 shallots (or 2 small onions), finely sliced
- 3 tsp fresh root ginger, grated or finely chopped
- 4 cm (1½ inches) galangal root, peeled and grated
- 2 red chillies, seeded and sliced
- 3 stalks lemongrass, smashed lightly and sliced
- 150 ml (5 fl oz) coconut cream
- 1 tbsp sunflower oil
- 1 tsp chilli powder
- 3 tsp turmeric
- 1 whole chicken, chopped into portions (your butcher will do this for you)
- 3 tbsp desiccated coconut, dry-fried on a medium-low heat until golden brown
- 1 tbsp brown sugar
- sea salt
- 3 kaffir lime leaves, torn up

Method

1. Put the shallots, ginger, galangal root, chillies and sliced lemongrass into a food processor, adding enough coconut cream to make a thick paste. If you don't have a food processor, grate all the ingredients and mix them with the coconut cream.

2. Heat the oil in a saucepan and stir-fry the shallot mix with the chilli powder, until soft but not browned, then add the turmeric and chicken pieces. Stir-fry for 5 minutes.

3. Add the rest of the coconut cream and the shallot paste. Cook on a medium heat until the curry thickens.

4. When the curry is thick and almost dry, add the fried desiccated coconut, brown sugar, salt and kaffir lime leaves. Allow everything to warm through as you stir it into the mix. Serve.

Therapeutic qualities

Chicken: Tonifies Qi.

Shallots, ginger, galangal, chillies, lime leaves, turmeric and lemongrass: Move Qi and prevent stagnation.

Coconut and brown sugar: Both tonify Qi and help harmonise the digestive system.

SPICY MACKEREL

Ingredients

- juice of 1 lime
- 1 tbsp fish sauce
- 1 tsp brown sugar
- 1 tbsp flavourless oil (groundnut oil works well)
- 2 sticks lemongrass, finely sliced
- 2 spring onions (scallions), finely sliced
- 1 red chilli, roughly chopped (ideally a hot chilli, like a Scotch bonnet)
- 2 cm (⅘ inch) fresh root ginger, grated or finely chopped
- small bunch coriander leaves (cilantro)
- 2 mackerel fillets

Method

1. Mix the lime juice with the fish sauce and brown sugar.

2. Heat the oil in a wok or frying pan and add the lemongrass, spring onions, chilli and ginger, and stir-fry briefly.

3. Pour the lime juice mixture into the wok, then scatter over the coriander leaves. Keep warm.

4. Grill or fry the mackerel fillets until cooked, add the stir-fried spices and serve.

Therapeutic qualities

Lemongrass, spring onions, chilli and ginger: All move Qi. Their warm nature mediates the cooling qualities of the lime and mackerel.

Coriander: Clears Empty Heat (a build-up of heat resulting from lack of Qi movement).

Lime: Its cooling astringent nature clears Heat.

Brown sugar: When combined with the lime it harmonises the digestive system.

Mackerel: Its cool, sweet nature clears Heat.

CHICKEN NOODLE SOUP

Ingredients

- 2 tsp red curry paste (see below)
- 1 chicken leg or breast
- 1½ litres (6 cups) chicken stock
- 100 g (3½ oz) rice noodles
- 1 red pepper (bell pepper), finely sliced
- 2 spring onions (scallions), finely sliced
- 3 tbsp parsley, chopped

RED CURRY PASTE

- 1 shallot (or small onion), finely chopped
- 1 stalk lemongrass, finely grated
- 1 tsp cayenne pepper
- 4 cloves garlic
- 2 cm (⅘ inch) fresh root ginger, sliced
- 2 tbsp tomato puree
- 3 tsp ground cumin
- 3 tsp ground coriander
- 3 tsp ground white pepper
- 2 tbsp soy sauce
- 1 tsp shrimp paste
- 1 tsp brown sugar
- 1 tbsp chilli powder
- 3 tbsp coconut milk
- 2 tbsp lime juice
- 1 tsp cinnamon

Method

1. Place all the ingredients for the curry paste in a food processor or blender and blend into a paste. If you don't have a food processor, grate all the ingredients and mix them with the coconut milk. This will produce enough paste to cover a full chicken. Freeze the mix in individual portions until you need it.

2. In a medium saucepan, bring the chicken and chicken stock to a simmer. Lower the heat, cover and simmer until the chicken is cooked through. Remove the chicken and shred the meat.

3. Whisk the curry paste into the stock and bring the stock back to a simmer. Add the noodles and red pepper and cook until the noodles are just tender. Stir in the chicken.

4. Serve garnished with spring onions and parsley.

Therapeutic qualities

Chicken: Qi tonic; its warm, sweet nature is comforting.

Pepper and spring onions: Move Qi, preventing stagnation.

Parsley: Regulates the flow of Qi.

Ginger, white pepper, lemongrass, shallots, cinnamon and chilli: All move Qi. Their warm nature mediates the cooling qualities of the soy sauce, coriander, tomato and lime.

Soy sauce and coriander: Clears Empty Heat (a build-up of heat resulting from lack of Qi movement).

Tomato and lime: Reinforce the Heat-clearing action of the soy sauce and coriander.

Cumin: Regulates the movement of Qi.

Shrimp paste and brown sugar: Are warm in nature; they tonify Qi while harmonising the digestive system.

ACUPRESSURE

How to apply pressure to the points

To press points, use something blunt. You can use finger pressure, but if you have to apply sustained pressure, you may find it uncomfortable. A chopstick (like the ones you get with a takeaway meal) is ideal for this purpose.

Ideally have someone do the treatment for you; that way you are not creating muscular tension while you try and reach points. You can also focus more on what sensations (or lack of them) result from pressing the point.

Don't press too hard; use enough pressure that you (or your partner) can feel something happening.

When you get to the point where something is happening, keep the pressure constant and hold for 30 seconds.

If you are not feeling any effects from pressing a point, you may not be pressing on the exact right spot. Try different spots around the location you first tried.

The points

There are any number of points that can be used, and in most cases points used in an acupuncture treatment are selected based on signs and symptoms presenting at that time. The points listed below are all useful in the treatment of PMS, but for a more individualised treatment plan, talk to a licensed acupuncture practitioner.

Points on the Liver Channel are particularly indicated in gynaecological conditions as both the main external portion of the Channel and a divergent branch strongly influence the genitalia, both internally and externally. In addition, the Liver's function of controlling the proper smooth flow of Qi means it can be useful in resolving many of the symptoms of PMS.

LIVER 3 (TAI CHONG) GREAT SURGE

Actions – Smooths the flow of Qi, nourishes Blood, regulates menstruation and regulates the lower abdominal and pelvic regions.

Location – On the dorsum of the foot in the depression distal to the junction of the first and second metatarsal bones.

Location note – Put your finger on the web between the big and second toe. Slide your finger upwards towards the ankle and you will find the junction of two bones. The point is in this junction.

LIVER 14 (QI MEN) CYCLE GATE

Actions – Regulates the flow of Qi and invigorates Blood.

Location – Directly below the nipple in the sixth intercostal space four finger breadths lateral to the anterior midline. In cases of Qi stagnation this point becomes very tender and easy to find.

GALL BLADDER 34 (YANG LING QUAN) YANG MOUND SPRING

Actions – Spreads Liver Qi and benefits the lateral costal region (the sides of the ribcage).

Location – In the depression approximately one finger breadth anterior and inferior to the head of the fibula.

Location note – Find your fibular head. This is a round bone just below the outside lower edge of your knee. Put your finger on the centre of this bone and then move it at a 45 degree angle forward – the hollow your finger falls into is the point.

SMALL INTESTINE 1 (SHAO ZE) LESSER MARSH

Actions – Benefits the breasts.

Location – Draw a line down from the outside edge of the nail of the little finger and another across the base; where they intersect is the point.

STOMACH 18 (RU GEN) BREAST ROOT

Actions – Benefits the breasts and reduces swelling; unbinds the chest.

Location – Directly below the nipple on the lower border of breast in the fifth intercostal space four finger breadths lateral to the anterior midline.

Location note – Directly below the midline of the breast, at the base of the breast.

This is a point combination that has proven very effective clinically as a basic protocol for any breast issue. Small Intestine 1 is the 'command point' of the breast – it controls the breast area via divergent Channels feeding off the Small Intestine main Channel.

Stomach 18 strongly affects not just the breast but also the intercostal muscles (between the ribs).

REFERENCES AND FURTHER READING

Chou, P. B., Morse, C. A. and Xu, H. (2008) 'A controlled trial of Chinese herbal medicine for premenstrual syndrome.' *Journal of Psychosomatic Obstetrics & Gynaecology 29*, 3, 185–192.

Freeman, E. W., Rickels, K., Yonkers, K. A. *et al.* (2001) 'Venlafaxine in the treatment of premenstrual dysphoric disorder.' *Obstetrics & Gynecology 98*, 737–744.

Guo, S. and Sun, Y. (2004) 'Comparison between acupuncture and medication in treatment of premenstrual syndrome.' *Shanghai Journal of Acupuncture and Moxibustion 23*, 5–6.

Jang, S. H., Kim, D. I. and Min-Sun Choi, M.-S. (2014) 'Effects and treatment methods of acupuncture and herbal medicine for premenstrual syndrome/premenstrual dysphoric disorder: Systematic review.' *BMC Complementary and Alternative Medicine 14*, I, II.

Johnson, J. A. (2000) *Chinese Medical Qigong Therapy: A Comprehensive Clinical Guide.* Pacific Grove, CA: International Institute of Medical Qigong.

Kwan, I. and Onwude, J. L. (1992) 'Premenstrual syndrome. Clinical evidence. Search date July 2009. Managing the premenstrual syndrome.' *Drug and Therapeutics Bulletin 30*, 69–72.

O'Brien, P. M. S. (1987) *Premenstrual Syndrome.* Oxford: Blackwell Scientific Publications.

O'Brien, P. M. S. (1993) 'Helping women with premenstrual syndrome.' *BMJ 307*, 1471–1475.

Rapkin, A. J., Morgan, M., Goldman, L. *et al.* (1997) 'Progesterone metabolite allopregnanolone in women with premenstrual syndrome.' *Obstetrics & Gynecology 90*, 709–714.

Sohrabi, N., Kashanian, M., Ghafoori, S. S. and Malakouti, S. K. (2013) 'Evaluation of the effect of omega-3 fatty acids in the treatment of premenstrual syndrome: A pilot trial.' *Complementary Therapies in Medicine*, June.

Steiner, M., Peer, M., Palova, E., Freeman, E. W., Macdougall, M. and Soares, C. N. (2011) 'The Premenstrual Symptoms Screening Tool revised for adolescents (PSST-A): Prevalence of severe PMS and premenstrual dysphoric disorder in adolescents.' *Archives of Women's Mental Health 14*, 1, 7–81.

Steiner, M., Romano, S. J., Babcock, S. *et al.* (2001) 'The efficacy of fluoxetine in improving physical symptoms associated with premenstrual dysphoric disorder.' *British Journal of Obstetrics & Gynaecology 108*, 462–468.

Wittchen, H.-U., Becker, E., Leib. R. and Krause, P. (2002) 'Prevalence, incidence and stability of premenstrual dysphoric disorder in the community.' *Psychiatric Medication 32*, 119–132.

Xu, Y. and Sun, Y. (2006) 'Observation of therapeutic effect of point-through-point acupuncture method in the back on premenstrual syndrome.' *Journal of Clinical Acupuncture and Moxibustion 22*, 37–38.

Chapter 13

MENOPAUSE

MENOPAUSE IN BIOMEDICINE

The medicalisation of menopause within biomedicine began in the early 19th century, and this has affected the way menopause is viewed, leading practitioners to think of menopause as a pathology. It may well be the case that diet and lifestyle in Asia is responsible for the lower incidence of menopausal symptoms. A colleague who specialises in the treatment of geriatric patients always emphasises that the best time to begin treating older people is when they are in their 20s, 30s and 40s. This is typical of the Chinese medicine approach – prevention is always better than cure. With a healthy diet and lifestyle, a problem is much less likely to manifest; this holds true as much for menopause as it does for anything else.

DIAGNOSIS OF MENOPAUSE

In most cases a diagnosis of menopause can be made based on menstrual history and current symptoms. In some cases blood tests are used to confirm the diagnosis.

Laboratory markers of menopause include the following:

- An increase in the serum follicle-stimulating hormone (FSH) and decreases in estradiol and inhibin are the major endocrine changes that occur during the transition to menopause.

- FSH levels are higher than luteinising hormone (LH) levels, and both rise to even higher values than those seen in the surge during the menstrual cycle.

COMMON SYMPTOMS

- Hot flushes: These are a sudden, transient sensation of warmth or heat that spreads over the body, creating a flushing, or redness, that is particularly noticeable on the face and upper body. Hot flushes result from a decreased supply of oestrogen, which occurs naturally as women approach menopause.

- Night sweats: For many women these are the most disruptive aspect of menopause, as a constantly interrupted sleep pattern can have knock-on implications for issues such as fatigue, mood swings or anxiety.

- Low libido: In menopausal women, the main cause of low sex drive is hormonal imbalance, in most cases an androgen deficiency. Other menopausal symptoms, such as vaginal dryness or depression, can also result in low libido.

- Vaginal dryness: As oestrogen levels drop during perimenopause, all skin becomes drier, thinner and less elastic. Vaginal tissue has a similar structure to all the other skin on your body, and as women get older, thinning of the skin of the vaginal wall can lead to dryness or, in some cases, atrophy (shrinking).

- Mood swings: These are caused primarily by hormonal imbalances; when production of oestrogen drops, so, too, does the production of mood-regulating neurotransmitters, resulting in mood swings. Other symptoms such as fatigue can also have a negative influence on mood.

- Anxiety: The hormone progesterone is involved with a calming neurotransmitter in the brain known as GABA (gamma-aminobutyric acid). As progesterone levels drop during perimenopause, it can lead to a reduced ability to manage stress and increased levels of anxiety. Issues such as sleep deprivation due to night sweats then add to the problem.

- Fatigue: Fatigue, one of the most common menopause symptoms, is caused by hormonal changes. Oestrogen (among other hormones) is used by the body to regulate energy use at a cellular level, so when oestrogen levels drop during menopause, so, too, do energy levels.

- Osteoporosis: This is a degenerative bone disorder, characterised by thinning and weakening of the bone and a general decrease in bone mass and density. Oestrogen is needed for calcium absorption into the bones, and because of the drop in oestrogen levels at perimenopause, women will experience an accelerated reduction in bone density from age 35 (approximately) onwards.

MENOPAUSE IN CHINESE MEDICINE

While Western medicine often views menopause as a disease, Chinese medicine recognises this change in a woman's body chemistry as a natural transitional process. It is unclear to what extent the various menopausal symptoms had been experienced by women in the Orient prior to the modern era. In Asia, women seeking treatment for conditions related to menopause are still a relative rarity; however, theories abound as to why this is, and most focus on diet and lifestyle. In the Western world underlying patterns of disharmony often give rise to the typical menopausal symptoms such as hot flushes, night sweats, headaches, mood swings, etc. Yin deficiency and resulting Heat and Dryness are typically the main issues.

VITAMIN AND MINERAL SUPPLEMENTS

For a full listing of the actions of common supplements according to Chinese medical theory, see Appendix B.

Although the best source of vitamins and minerals is through a well-balanced diet, many foods today are lacking in these vital trace elements. A point I always try and stress to people is that cheap supplements are cheap for a reason. Discount supplements often use raw ingredients that are low quality and have a poor level of absorption.

Vitamin B6: Reduces homocysteine levels. Homocysteine is an amino acid associated with increased risk of heart attack and impairment of bone formation.

Vitamin C: Helps to build up collagen reserves. Collagen is a major building block of both bone and connective tissue.

Vitamin D: Increases calcium absorption.

Vitamin E: Hormone replacement therapy (HRT) has been shown to increase the risk of heart attacks and strokes, but a recent study (see EBCTCG 2015) showed a 75 per cent reduction in the risk of heart attack with vitamin E supplementation.

Vitamin K: Plays a role in bone calcification.

Boron: Helps calcium absorption by the bones, and may potentiate the action of oestrogen.

Calcium: Hydroxyapatite (derived from bone), calcium citrate and calcium malate are currently thought to be the best sources for preventing and treating osteoporosis. Aside from bone health, calcium is essential for the proper functioning of the nervous system.

Folic acid: Reduces the build-up of homocysteine, an amino acid associated with increased risk of heart attack and impairment of bone formation.

Magnesium: Current recommendations are to consume at least half as much magnesium as calcium. Magnesium enhances calcium absorption and retention. Magnesium acts as a natural tranquilliser and can help prevent or treat anxiety.

Manganese: Necessary for bone mineralisation.

Silicon: Aids calcium absorption into bone and adds structural strength to bones, ligaments and tendons.

Zinc: Necessary for bone formation; it also increases vitamin D activity and promotes immune functions.

THERAPEUTIC RECIPES

For a complete listing of the energetic qualities and uses in Chinese medicine of most common foods, see Appendix A.

Breakfast

Porridge made with water and sprinkled with cinnamon. Porridge is warming in nature; it improves digestive function and Blood circulation. Cinnamon improves Blood circulation in the smaller vessels such as those in the fingers, toes or around the reproductive organs.

Walnuts and/or cashews in natural yoghurt. Although yoghurt is considered cold in nature, both walnuts and cashews are warming. It is important to choose yoghurt with no added sugar and live bacteria.

Lunch

Salad: Many salad vegetables are cold in nature (this can slow down digestive function and impair the movement of Qi and Blood), but the addition of onions, garlic, ginger, chilli or peppers can mediate the cooling action of the vegetables.

Try some of the following combinations:

Carrot, apple and ginger

Carrot and radish

Duck, watercress and orange

Guacamole

Mixed beans with chilli

Prawns with bean sprouts

Dinner

BEEF STEW WITH BONE BROTH

Ingredients

- 300 g (10 oz) beef bones (shin is ideal – you can get shin beef on the bone from a butcher)
- 100 g (3½ oz) stewing beef, cubed
- 50 g (2 oz) goji berries
- 1 tbsp apple cider vinegar
- 2 carrots, chopped
- 1 leek, sliced
- 40 g (2 oz) pearl barley

Method

1. Put all the ingredients into a pot and cover with water.
2. Bring to a boil and simmer for 1.5–2 hours.
3. Serve.

Therapeutic qualities

Beef bones: Nourish Yin and Blood. Everything needed for good bone health is contained in the soup bones.

Beef: Nourishes Qi and Blood.

Goji berries: Nourish Yin and Blood.

Apple cider vinegar: Helps the nutrients leach out of the bones into the broth.

Carrot: Nourishes Yin.

Leek: Tonifies Yang; all the other ingredients strongly nourish Yin, and without the leek to move Qi, the recipe could be too cloying, resulting in Dampness (fluid stagnation).

Pearl barley: This prevents an accumulation of assimilated fluids that would lead to a condition of Dampness.

KIWIFRUIT AND AVOCADO SALAD

Ingredients

- 2 kiwifruit, peeled and sliced
- 2 avocados, peeled and sliced
- 100 g (3½ oz) grapes, sliced in half
- 100 g (3½ oz) spinach leaves
- 2 tsp balsamic vinegar

Method

1. Arrange the kiwifruit, avocado, grapes and spinach leaves in individual serving bowls.

2. Dress with the balsamic vinegar and serve.

Therapeutic qualities

Kiwifruit: Clears Heat and nourishes Body Fluids.

Avocado: Clears Heat and nourishes Body Fluids.

Grapes: Qi and Blood tonics.

Spinach: Traditionally prescribed to treat hypertension, it has a cool nature. Spinach is rich in oxalic acid that decreases the absorption of calcium, so avoid eating it if you suffer from osteoporosis or similar diseases causing lack of calcium.

Balsamic vinegar: Its sour nature and astringent qualities help to clear Heat.

 SALMON CURRY

Ingredients

- red curry paste (see below)
- 100 g (3½ oz) pearl barley
- olive oil
- 2 cloves garlic, grated or finely chopped
- 1 tsp fresh root ginger, grated or finely chopped
- 400 ml (14 fl oz) coconut milk
- 1 lemon, zest and juice
- 2 salmon steaks
- 1 stalk celery, sliced
- 2 spring onions (scallions), finely sliced

RED CURRY PASTE

- 1 stalk lemongrass, roughly chopped
- 1 small shallot, grated
- 1 clove garlic, grated or finely chopped
- 1 tsp galangal (or fresh root ginger), grated or finely chopped
- 1 tsp coriander seeds
- 1 lime leaf, shredded
- 1 tsp ground cumin
- 2 tbsp groundnut oil
- sea salt

Method

1. Blend all the ingredients for the red curry paste.
2. Cook the pearl barley in boiling salted water, and set it aside.
3. In the same pot used to cook the barley, heat 2 teaspoons of oil, add the garlic and ginger and cook until fragrant.
4. Add the red curry paste and pearl barley.
5. Stir in the coconut milk and lemon zest (and water if needed to loosen the mix) and add the salmon, celery and spring onions.
6. Reduce the heat to low, and cook until the flavours are thoroughly combined.

Therapeutic qualities

Salmon: Nourishes Yin and builds Body Fluids and the ability to cool and lubricate.

Lemon: Clears Heat and helps retain Body Fluids.

Coconut milk: Tonifies Qi while it nourishes Yin.

Lemongrass, shallots, galangal, lime leaf, chilli, garlic, spring onions and onion: All move Qi. Their warm nature mediates the cooling qualities of the salmon and coconut milk.

Coriander: Clears Empty Heat (a build-up of heat resulting from lack of Qi movement).

Cumin: Regulates the movement of Qi.

Pearl barley and celery: Drains any Dampness (stagnant fluid) caused by the cloying damp nature of some of the ingredients.

BRAISED PORK BELLY

Ingredients

- 1 tbsp butter
- 200 g (7 oz) pork belly, skin removed
- 1 litre (4 cups) vegetable stock
- 1 onion, chopped
- 1 stick celery, chopped
- 1 large carrot, peeled and chopped
- 3 tsp honey
- sea salt and black pepper

Method

1. Melt the butter in a heavy-bottomed pan. Add the pork belly, fat side down, and cook until the fat is brown.

2. Add the other ingredients, cover with the vegetable stock and cook on a medium heat until the pork is cooked.

3. Remove the vegetables and strain before pouring the liquid back over the pork.

4. Serve with steamed rice or green vegetables.

Therapeutic qualities

Pork: Nourishes Yin, the body's innate ability to cool and moisten itself.

Butter, carrot and honey: All enhance the Yin tonifying qualities of the pork.

Onion: Moves Qi and prevents the other ingredients causing stagnation or a build-up of fluids.

Celery: Drains any Dampness (stagnant fluid) caused by the cloying damp nature of some of the ingredients.

GRILLED CHICKEN SALAD WITH AVOCADO AND MANGO

Ingredients

- 4 tsp soy sauce
- 3 tbsp lime juice
- 1 tsp fresh root ginger, grated or finely chopped
- 1 chicken breast, grilled and sliced
- 1 mango, diced
- 1 avocado, diced
- lettuce

Method

1. To make the dressing, combine the soy sauce with the lime juice and ginger.
2. When the chicken is cool, combine it with the mango, avocado and lettuce, and pour over the dressing. Serve.

Therapeutic qualities

Chicken: Qi tonic (energy levels are often an issue during menopause).

Soy sauce: Clears Heat.

Lettuce, mango, lime juice and avocado: Clear Heat; lettuce also has a calming effect.

Ginger: Moves Qi and Body Fluids; its warm nature mediates the cooling nature of the other ingredients.

FISH STEW

Ingredients

- 1 tbsp olive oil
- 2 cloves garlic, grated or finely chopped
- 2 tsp turmeric
- 100 g (3½ oz) tomatoes, peeled
- 100 g (3½ oz) adzuki beans
- 2 mackerel fillets (any oily fish will work)
- handful of coriander (cilantro)

Method

1. Heat the olive oil in a large saucepan over a medium heat. Add the garlic and turmeric. Cook, stirring, for 30 seconds.

2. Reduce the heat to low. Stir in the tomatoes and 284 ml (1 cup) of cold water. Cover and bring to the boil. Simmer, covered, for 10 minutes.

3. Add the beans and return to the boil. Add the fish. Cover and cook until the fish is cooked through.

4. Serve garnished with coriander.

Therapeutic qualities

Oily fish such as mackerel: Nourish Yin and help prevent inflammation.

Tomatoes: Clear Heat and produce Body Fluids.

Adzuki beans: Clear Heat and drain Dampness (stagnant fluids).

Turmeric: Has anti-inflammatory qualities and helps clear Heat.

Garlic: Provides some warmth to balance out the overall cooling nature of the dish.

 ## HONEY-GLAZED PORK

Ingredients

- 1 tbsp Dijon mustard
- 2 tbsp honey
- 2 small cloves garlic, grated or finely chopped
- 2 tsp rosemary, chopped
- lemon zest
- black pepper
- 1 pork chop

Method

1. Combine the mustard, honey, garlic, rosemary and lemon zest in a bowl. Season with the pepper.

2. Add the pork and coat it well. Cover with plastic wrap. Place in the fridge to marinate (ideally overnight).

3. Heat the oven to 190°C/Gas Mark 6/375°F.

4. Place the pork on a roasting rack and reserve the marinade. Bake on a medium heat until cooked through.

5. Put the reserved marinade in a small saucepan over a medium heat. Bring to the boil and cook until it thickens slightly.

6. Drizzle the marinade over rice or vegetables to accompany the pork.

Therapeutic qualities

Pork: Nourishes Yin, the body's innate ability to cool and moisten itself.

Honey and lemon zest: Honey has a cooling moistening quality that is mediated by the Qi-moving qualities of the lemon zest.

Dijon mustard and garlic: Move Qi. Their warming natures are counterbalanced by the pork, honey and rosemary.

Rosemary: Recent research has shown that rosemary can help prevent age-related skin damage. The two key ingredients in rosemary – caffeic acid and rosemarinic acid – are potent antioxidant and anti-inflammatory agents.

 YAM AND PINEAPPLE CASSEROLE

Ingredients

- 1 yam, peeled
- 60 g (2 oz) pineapple
- 2 tsp cinnamon
- 1 tbsp ground flaxseed

Method

1. Cook the yam in a large pot of salted water until tender.

2. Dice the yam and place in a baking dish.

3. Stir the pineapple, cinnamon and flaxseed into the casserole dish.

4. Preheat the oven to 175°C/Gas Mark 4/350°F.

5. Place the casserole dish in the oven and bake for 35 minutes. Serve.

Therapeutic qualities

Yam: Tonifies Qi and produces Body Fluids.

Pineapple: Clears Heat and produces Body Fluids.

Flaxseed: Nourishes Yin.

Cinnamon: The gentle warmth of cinnamon moves Qi and Body Fluids, thus preventing them stagnating. It also mediates the cold nature of the other ingredients.

ACUPRESSURE

How to apply pressure to the points

To press points, use something blunt. You can use finger pressure, but if you have to apply sustained pressure, you may find it uncomfortable. A chopstick (like the ones you get with a takeaway meal) is ideal for this purpose.

Ideally have someone do the treatment for you; that way you are not creating muscular tension while you try and reach points. You can also focus more on what sensations (or lack of them) result from pressing the point.

Don't press too hard; use enough pressure that you (or your partner) can feel something happening.

When you get to the point where something is happening, keep the pressure constant and hold for 30 seconds.

If you are not feeling any effects from pressing a point, you may not be pressing on the exact right spot. Try different spots around the location you first tried.

The points

There are any number of points that can be used, and in most cases points used in an acupuncture treatment are selected based on signs and symptoms presenting at that time. The points listed below are all useful, but for a more individualised treatment plan, talk to a licensed acupuncture practitioner.

HEART 3 (SHAO HAI) LESSER SEA

Actions – Calms the mind and clears Heat.

Location – With the elbow flexed, at the midpoint of the line connecting the medial end of the cubital crease and the medial epicondyle of humerus.

Location note – The point is in the soft flesh on the inside of the elbow, just off the bone.

HEART 6 (YIN XI) YIN CLEFT

Actions – Stops night sweating and calms the mind.

Location – When the palm faces upward, the point is on the radial side of the tendon of the flexor carpi ulnaris muscle, one finger breadth above the transverse crease of the wrist.

Location note – The point is on the inside of your wrist crease (little finger side). At the base of your hand where it joins the wrist there is a round bone (pisiform). The point is one finger breadth up on the inside edge of the tendon (that stringy structure you will feel as you press on the wrist).

TRIPLE WARMER 2 (YE MEN) HUMOUR GATE

Actions – Disperses Heat and calms the mind.

Location – When the fist is clenched, the point is located on the margin of the web between the ring and small fingers at the junction of the red and white skin.

KIDNEY 2 (RAN GU) BLAZING VALLEY

Actions – Clears Empty Heat and regulates the Kidneys.

Location – Anterior and inferior to the medial malleolus, in the depression on the lower border of the tuberosity of the navicular bone.

Location note – As you look down at your foot (inside edge), there is a bump just in front of your ankle – this is the navicular bone.

KIDNEY 6 (ZHAO HAI) SHINING SEA

Actions – Nourishes the Kidneys, clears Empty Heat and calms the mind.

Location – In the depression below the tip of the medial malleolus.

Location note – Put your finger on the round bone that sticks out from your inner ankle; now let your finger drop straight down. The little groove your finger falls into is the point.

GALL BLADDER 39 (XUAN ZHONG) SUSPENDED BELL

Actions – Benefits the sinews and the bones.

Location – Three finger breadths above the tip of the external malleolus on the anterior border of the fibula.

BLADDER 40 (WEI ZHONG) EQUILIBRIUM MIDDLE

Actions – Clears Heat.

Location – Midpoint of the transverse crease of the popliteal fossa between the tendons of the biceps femoris and semitendinosus muscles.

Location note – The point is on the midpoint of the crease at the back of the knee. Don't press too deeply as there is an artery directly below.

REFERENCES AND FURTHER READING

Adashi, E. Y. (1994) 'The climacteric ovary as a functional gonadotropin-driven androgen-producing gland.' *Fertility and Sterility 62*, 20–27.

Collaborative Group on Epidemiological Studies of Ovarian Cancer (2015) 'Menopausal hormone use and ovarian cancer risk: Individual participant meta-analysis of 52 epidemiological studies.' *The Lancet*. doi: 10.1016/S0140-6736(14)61687-1

EBCTCG (Early Breast Cancer Trialists' Collaborative Group) (2015) 'Aromatase inhibitors versus tamoxifen in early breast cancer: Patient-level meta-analysis of the randomised trials.' *The Lancet 386*, 10001, 1341–1352.

Furth, C. A. (1999) *Flourishing Yin: Gender in China's Medical History, 960–1665.* Berkeley, CA: University of California Press.

GISSI (Gruppo Italiano per lo Studio della Sopravvivenza nell'Infarto miocardico) (1999) 'Dietary supplementation with n-3 polyunsaturated fatty acids and vitamin E after myocardial infarction: Results of the GISSI-Prevenzione trial. Gruppo Italiano per lo Studio della Sopravvivenza nell'Infarto miocardico.' *The Lancet 354*, 447–455.

Hercberg, S., Galan, P., Preziosi, P. *et al.* (2004) 'The SU.VI.MAX Study: A randomized, placebo-controlled trial of the health effects of antioxidant vitamins and minerals.' *Archives of Internal Medicine 164*, 2335–2342.

Hunter, D. J., Manson, J. E., Colditz, G. A. *et al.* (1993) 'A prospective study of the intake of vitamins C, E, and A and the risk of breast cancer.' *New England Journal of Medicine 329*, 234–240.

Kang, H. S., Jeong, D., Kim, D. I. and Lee, M. S. (2011) 'The use of acupuncture for managing gynaecologic conditions: An overview of systematic reviews.' *Maturitas 68*, 4, 346–354.

Langevin, H. M., Wayne, P. M., Macpherson, H. *et al.* (2011) 'Paradoxes in acupuncture research: Strategies for moving forward.' *Evidence-Based Complementary and Alternative Medicine*, volume 2011, article ID 180805.

Li, L. (1994) 'Clinical observation on osteoporosis treated with traditional kidney-tonifying medicaments.' *Journal of Traditional Chinese Medicine 14*, 1, 41–44.

Petti, F., Bangrazi, A., Liguori, A., Reale, G. and Ippoliti, F. (1998) 'Effects of acupuncture on immune response related to opioid-like peptides.' *Journal of Traditional Chinese Medicine 18*, 1, 55–63.

Stampfer, M. J., Hennekens, C. H., Manson, J. E., Colditz, G. A., Rosner, B. and Willett, W. C. (1993) 'Vitamin E consumption and the risk of coronary disease in women.' *New England Journal of Medicine 328*, 1444–1449.

Stener-Victorin, E., Fujisawa, S. and Kurosawa, M. (1985) 'Ovarian blood flow responses to electroacupuncture stimulation depend on estrous cycle and on site and frequency of stimulation in anesthetized rats.' *Journal of Applied Physiology 101*, 1, 84–91.

Stener-Victorin, E., Waldenström, U., Andersson, S. A. and Wikland, M. (1996) 'Reduction of blood flow impedance in the uterine arteries of infertility women with electro-acupuncture.' *Human Reproduction 11*, 6, 1314–1317.

Yuankai, L. Songping, L., Yuzhen, Z. and Guozhen, L. (1989) 'Menopause syndrome treated by traditional Chinese medicine.' *Journal of the American College of Traditional Chinese Medicine 7*, 1–2, 55–64.

Chapter 14

ASSISTED REPRODUCTIVE TECHNOLOGY

Assisted reproductive technology (ART) is the branch of medicine that specialises in helping couples who are experiencing problems conceiving. The original technology was developed in the 1970s, and in 1978 the first baby conceived 'in vitro' (literally, 'in glass') was born.

IN VITRO FERTILISATION

Mental preparation for in vitro fertilisation

In vitro fertilisation (IVF) has the potential to be an emotionally, physically and financially exhausting experience, and emotional preparation for an IVF cycle is as important as preparing yourself physically. Your mental and physical health are intertwined, and any adverse change in one can affect the other too.

Patients have rated the stress of undergoing IVF as more stressful than or almost as stressful as any other major life event that they have experienced. Stress can mean many things, and each person will experience stress differently based on their own personality and life experiences. If you ask the next one hundred people you meet, 'What does stress mean to you?', you will get a hundred different answers, as each body/mind combination reacts in an individual way. It is important to recognise the effects of stress not only in yourself but also in your partner; in doing so couples can learn coping skills and communication patterns that will enable them to support each other through the IVF cycle and beyond.

Can the mind influence the body?

It is a proven scientific reality that the mind and body are interactive and constantly influence and affect each other. (This relatively new field of medicine is called psychoneuroimmunology.)

> Our physical body can be changed by the emotions we experience. (Pert 1999)

In clinic I have seen patients where prolonged periods of stress led to complete suppression of their menstrual cycle. There was nothing physically 'wrong'; it was an emotion that shut down the production of or distribution of the hormones needed for a period to occur. There are many diseases with no known organic cause to be found in medical literature; for example, irritable bowel syndrome, where the symptoms are plain to see but there is nothing physically wrong, no bacteria, no virus, nothing that can be put under a microscope, but yet there is illness.

Dr John Upledger (founder of craniosacral therapy) frequently refers to 'somato emotional cysts' in his textbooks (see Upledger 1997). He describes these cysts as failures and disappointments that are ignored and left to fester. We know that issues with conceiving can affect work, friendships, family and relationships.

What this means for you going into an IVF cycle is that you need to be aware that only about 40 per cent of IVF cycles end in pregnancy. Going through the IVF cycle hoping and praying that you are going to be in that 40 per cent can leave you devastated if, after everything, there is a negative pregnancy test. On the other hand, if you are totally pessimistic from the outset, just imagine what sort of signals your body is receiving from your mind. So, as with everything in life, moderation is key – don't let the IVF take over your whole life; make time to have fun and enjoy life.

What you can do

- The first treatment cycle is typically the most stressful for patients. With the possibility of high levels of confusion and anxiety, one of the best antidotes for anxiety associated with a first-time IVF cycle is information and knowledge. Being knowledgeable about the medications and treatment protocols can help make you feel less of a spectator and more of a player in the entire IVF process.

- Plan ahead. It is important to anticipate decisions that you may have to make during an IVF cycle and discuss your options ahead of time.

- Decide which of your friends and family you are going to tell that you are going to try IVF. You need support and encouragement, not constant questioning about IVF protocols or drug side effects.

- Online support groups may provide this support if friends and family cannot. Even in cases where you have supportive friends and family, online support groups can provide insights that only someone going through the IVF process can give you.

- Decide what you have control over and what you don't. Eliminate any unnecessary stress and make your life as simple as possible during the cycle. This is not a time to make important decisions or changes in your life, such as moving house or job.

- If you do not have a hobby before you begin IVF, find one. You need to have something to occupy your body and mind totally separate from anything to do with IVF. This is time for you, where all you need to focus on is your chosen hobby, whatever it is.

- Begin to learn relaxation techniques either on DVD or, better still, in a class before you begin IVF. There's no point trying to learn to relax after you're stressed with all the new medical jargon, blood tests, injections and scans.

- Constant negative pregnancy tests may have taken a toll on how you are feeling about yourself, your marital relationship and your relationship with friends and family, causing distress and isolation. You will want to be in a good place emotionally and have your relationships on solid ground before starting an IVF cycle.

Typical protocol for in vitro fertilisation

If you are planning IVF, the protocol will vary a little from clinic to clinic and adjustments may have to be made to suit your personal circumstances, but the basics remain the same, and a typical protocol is laid out below.

- Oral contraceptive pills: Oral contraceptive pills can be used to begin taking control of your cycle. Even if your cycle is regular, the timing of a natural period may not suit the hospital timetable.

- GnRH antagonist administration: You will usually begin treatment with a GnRH antagonist on approximately the sixteenth day of taking oral contraceptive pills (or around day six, if you are taking progesterone).

- Baseline pelvic ultrasound: Around day one of your period, the clinic will perform an ultrasound scan to examine the condition of your ovaries. A blood test (serum estradiol (E2) measurement) to confirm that the ovaries are properly suppressed can be done at the same time.

- Ovarian stimulation: Ovarian stimulation can begin after menstrual bleeding starts. This is generally done by self-administered intramuscular injection.

- Monitoring of follicle development: Follicular (egg) development can be assessed by measuring blood hormone (estradiol) levels or a vaginal ultrasound. Testing is typically done every three days so that the dosage of medications can be altered as needed as excessive follicular growth can lead to ovarian hyperstimulation syndrome (OHSS), a potentially serious condition.

- Egg maturation: Human chorionic gonadotropin (hCG) is the hormone that is used to stimulate the final maturation of your eggs. Determining the proper day for hCG administration is critical. If it is administered too early, few, if any, eggs will be mature. If it is administered too late, the eggs within the follicles may be post-mature (atretic) and will not fertilise. Optimal egg maturity occurs when follicles measure at least 18-20 mm (0.7-0.8 inches) and serum estradiol is greater than 2000 pg/mL.

- Egg retrieval: Typically egg retrieval is performed about 34-36 hours after hCG has been administered. The number of eggs retrieved is related to the number of follicles present, their accessibility and the number of follicles that develop in response to stimulation. Ultrasound provides only an approximation of the number of eggs that one can expect to recover. At this stage of proceedings remember that, no matter how many eggs are retrieved, they probably won't all develop into viable embryos, and not all of the embryos that develop will be suitable for transfer.

- Insemination: Laboratory staff will examine the fluid aspirated from your follicles for the presence of eggs. Not every follicle contains an egg, and rarely, a follicle may contain more than one. The semen specimen is prepared using techniques designed to separate the sperm from other material present in the ejaculate. The most active sperm are placed in a culture dish with an egg. The dish is placed into an incubator that maintains a specific temperature, pH, level of humidity and concentration of carbon dioxide. After 12-20 hours it will be possible to detect evidence of fertilisation under the microscope.

- Embryo transfer: The embryo transfer procedure is usually performed three to five days after egg retrieval. The procedure is nearly identical to that used in intrauterine insemination. A catheter is passed through the cervix into the uterus and deposits the embryos into the uterine cavity along with an extremely small amount of fluid.

- Progesterone supplements: Progesterone helps prepare the uterine lining for implantation, and it is important that progesterone levels remain high throughout the early stages of a pregnancy.

- Pregnancy test: A serum pregnancy test is normally done 12-14 days after the embryo transfer, and all being well, the result will be positive. In some cases the standard

IVF protocol will not prove successful or there may be limiting factors that make a standard protocol impossible (for example, very low sperm quality). In these cases other specialised procedures such as intracytoplasmic sperm injection (ICSI), a process where a sperm is literally injected into the egg, may be used.

INTRAUTERINE INSEMINATION

Intrauterine insemination (IUI) is one of the least invasive ART procedures, and as such poses relatively few risks for the patient. It is often explored as a treatment option before going on to IVF. In some cases IUI can be used as part of a normal menstrual cycle with no need for drugs to induce ovarian stimulation. The reasons for doing this can include:

- Male factors: Your partner's semen analysis may show problems such as sperm motility, shape or count. IUI can overcome these problems because sperm are washed and separated from the other components within the semen, and then the best quality, most motile sperm are selected for insemination; basically they are given a head start that should help overcome any of the difficulties mentioned.

- Unexplained sub-fertility: IUI is often used as a first treatment for unexplained sub-fertility as it is relatively non-invasive.

- Cervical hostility: The mucus produced by the cervix around the time of ovulation is supposed to provide an ideal environment for sperm to travel from the vagina to the fallopian tubes; however, if the cervical mucus is too thick, or too acidic, it may trap or kill sperm before they reach the uterus. IUI avoids this problem by bypassing the cervix and depositing the sperm directly into the uterus. A cheap acid/alkaline test strip is available from any pharmacy.

- Donor sperm: For people who need to use donor sperm to get pregnant, IUI can be used to achieve pregnancy.

IUI success rates vary widely from clinic to clinic, but there are four major factors to take into account:

- Maternal age. Ovarian reserve and egg quality are both directly linked to age, and as you age the quality of your eggs and their ability to fertilise and develop normally diminishes (see the 'Diminished ovarian reserve' section in Chapter 7).

- The cause of the sub-fertility. In cases of unexplained sub-fertility where no organic cause is found, there is a reasonably good chance of success, but other common conditions such as endometriosis may lessen your chances.

- The quality of the sperm available. Clinical studies have shown that IUI can be effective for some couples where poor sperm quality is the key factor. However, there are limits to what can be achieved with IUI. If the total motile sperm count at the time of insemination (after the processing) is less than 5 million, the chances for pregnancy are small. If the total motile sperm count is below 1 to 5 million, success rates are substantially lower, and IVF may be a better option.

- Any degree of tubal damage or pelvic scarring (see Chapter 7).

CAFFEINE AND ALCOHOL

Over the last number of years there has been conflicting advice on both caffeine and alcohol consumption both pre-conception and during pregnancy. Medical research carried out over the last decade has produced some interesting results.

Caffeine and pre-eclampsia

Moderate caffeine consumption may actually have a preventative function in relation to pre-eclampsia. A Dutch study (Bakker *et al.* 2011) found that 'Higher caffeine intake during pregnancy seems to be associated with elevated systolic blood pressure levels in first and third trimester, but not with diastolic blood pressure levels.

We did not find evidence of significant adverse associations of caffeine intake on maternal cardiovascular adaptations during pregnancy.' Put simply, caffeine doesn't cause elevated blood pressure or contribute to pre-eclampsia.

Caffeine and miscarriage

Danish researchers questioned more than 80,000 pregnant women regarding their coffee intake. This study found that women who drank large amounts of coffee during pregnancy were more likely to experience a miscarriage. Women who drank more than two cups of coffee a day had a slightly increased risk of miscarriage, while those who drank eight or more cups experienced a 59 per cent increase in miscarriage (see Bech *et al.* 2005).

Caffeine and the time taken to conceive

A study conducted at Yale University School of Medicine does seem to add credence to the theory that excessive caffeine intake can affect the amount of time it takes to conceive. The researchers found that 'women who reported drinking over 300 mg/day of caffeine had a 27% lower chance of conceiving for each cycle, and those who reported drinking less than 300 mg/day had a 10% reduction in per cycle conception rates' (Hatch and Bracken 1993).

Caffeine, final thoughts

Large-scale studies conducted over the last decade have shown no association between birth defects and caffeine consumption; however, caffeine easily passes from mother to foetus through the placenta. Adults have fully developed systems for breaking down and eliminating chemicals (such as caffeine), but these systems are not fully developed in an unborn child, and blood levels of caffeine may remain elevated for longer periods in the unborn child compared to the mother.

Some reports have stated that children born to mothers who consumed more than 500 mg of caffeine a day were more likely to have faster heart rates, tremors, an increased breathing rate and spend more time awake in the days following birth.

Alcohol

Alcohol was confirmed as a teratogen (an agent or influence that causes physical defects in the developing embryo) in the late 1970s after observations made in France and the US in infants born to alcoholic mothers. Everyone knows the damaging effects of consuming excessive amounts of alcohol in pregnancy; however, there is a lack of consensus regarding what constitutes excessive drinking. The best option may be to follow the advice given in the *British Medical Journal*:

> Pregnant women and women planning to become pregnant should be advised to abstain from drinking, as even those women who adhered to the UK guidelines of 1–2 units once or twice a week in the first trimester were at risk of having babies with reduced birth weight and born preterm when compared to mothers who abstained from alcohol. (Mathews, Yudkin and Neil 1999)

Male fertility can be severely compromised by over-consumption of alcohol (approximately 80 per cent of male alcoholics are sterile). Alcohol can affect male fertility in the following ways:

- Acetaldehyde, a breakdown byproduct of alcohol metabolism, is highly toxic to sperm.

- Alcohol consumption can increase the number of sperm abnormalities.

- Alcohol consumption can lead to chromosomal abnormalities within sperm.

- Alcohol can affect sperm motility.

VITAMIN AND MINERAL SUPPLEMENTS

The best way to be sure you are getting all these nutrients into you (and your partner) is to eat a varied diet. Unfortunately, with nutritional deficiencies in the soil, food grown will not always ensure you are getting all you need. In this case, a good multi-mineral and vitamin supplement is required (talk to your local pharmacist or health food shop).

Vitamin A: Has strong antioxidant properties and is vital for the production of female sex hormones.

Vitamin B1 (thiamine): Deficiency of B1 can lead to failed ovulation or implantation.

Vitamin B2 (riboflavin): Deficiencies of B2 have been linked to miscarriage and low birth weight.

Vitamin B3 (niacin): Important for sex hormone production.

Vitamin B5: Important for foetal development.

Vitamin B6: Together with zinc, B6 is vital for the development and proper utilisation of oestrogen and progesterone.

Vitamin B9 (folate; folic acid): Reduces the risk of neural tube defects in your baby.

Vitamin B12: Needed for the synthesis of DNA and RNA.

Vitamin C: Antioxidant. Take care with doses exceeding 1000 mg a day as this can have an antihistamine effect and dry up cervical mucus.

Vitamin E: Deficiency has been linked to irregular ovulation and miscarriage.

Vitamin K: Essential for blood clotting.

Calcium: Essential for hormonal balance.

Chromium: Needed for the regulation of hormone and blood sugar levels.

Iron: Deficiency is very common and can lead to miscarriage.

Magnesium: Deficiencies have been linked to female infertility.

Manganese: Deficiencies can lead to impaired ovarian function.

Selenium: Deficiencies have been linked to female infertility.

Zinc: Essential as a co-factor in hundreds of enzyme reactions. Deficiency can cause a vast range of symptoms.

ACUPRESSURE

How to apply pressure to the points

To press points, use something blunt. You can use finger pressure, but if you have to apply sustained pressure, you may find it uncomfortable. A chopstick (like the ones you get with a takeaway meal) is ideal for this purpose.

Ideally have someone do the treatment for you; that way you are not creating muscular tension while you try and reach points. You can also focus more on what sensations (or lack of them) result from pressing the point.

Don't press too hard; use enough pressure that you (or your partner) can feel something happening.

When you get to the point where something is happening, keep the pressure constant and hold for 30 seconds.

If you are not feeling any effects from pressing a point, you may not be pressing on the exact right spot. Try different spots around the location you first tried.

The points

There are any number of points that can be used, and in most cases points used in an acupuncture treatment are selected based on signs and symptoms presenting at that time. The points listed below are all useful, but for a more individualised treatment plan, talk to a licensed acupuncture practitioner.

These points can cause a very strong ovarian response:

- Do not stimulate them unless there is a poor response to your drug regime.

- Do not stimulate these points for more than three days at a time without checking ovarian function.

- If you notice any premenstrual-type bloating, stop stimulating the points.

REN 1 (HUI YIN) MEETING OF YIN

Actions – Combines with Zi Gong Xue (extra point below) to stimulate ovarian function when there is no response to ovarian stimulation.

Location – Between the anus and the posterior labial commissure.

REN 3 (ZHONG JI) CENTRAL POLE

Actions – Benefits the uterus and fortifies the Kidneys.

Location – On the anterior midline four finger breadths below the umbilicus.

REN 4 (GUAN YUAN) ORIGIN PASS MEETING

Actions – Benefits the uterus and assists conception.

Location – On the anterior midline four finger breadths below the umbilicus.

REN 5 (SHI MEN) STONE GATE

Actions – Regulates the uterus.

Location – On the anterior midline two finger breadths below the umbilicus.

KIDNEY 1 (YONG QUAN) BUBBLING WELL

Actions – When combined with Zi Gong Xue (see below), stimulates ovarian function.

Location – On the sole of the foot, approximately at the junction of the anterior one-third and posterior two-thirds of the line connecting the base of the second and third toes and the heel.

Location note – Divide the sole of the foot into thirds. The point is on the line dividing the middle and top third, in the centre of the line.

ZI GONG XUE (EYES OF THE OVARIES)

Actions – Stimulates ovarian function.

Location – Four finger breadths down from the navel and five finger breadths from the midline.

REFERENCES AND FURTHER READING

Bailey, B. A. and Sokol, R. J. (2011) 'Prenatal alcohol exposure and miscarriage, stillbirth, preterm delivery, and sudden infant death syndrome.' *Alcohol Research & Health 34*, 1, 86–91.

Bakker, R., Steegers, E. A., Raat, H., Hofman, A. and Jaddoe, V. W. (2011) 'Maternal caffeine intake, blood pressure, and the risk of hypertensive complications during pregnancy: The Generation R Study.' *American Journal of Hypertension 24*, 4, 421–428.

Bech, B. H., Nohr, E. A., Vaeth, M., Henriksen, T. B. and Olsen, J. (2005) 'Coffee and fetal death: A cohort study with prospective data.' *American Journal of Epidemiology 162*, 10, 983–990.

Broderick, J. E. (2000) 'Mind-body medicine in rheumatologic disease.' *Rheumatic Disease Clinics of North America 26*, 1, 161–176.

Clausson, B., Granath, F., Ekbom, A. *et al.* (2002) 'Effect of caffeine exposure during pregnancy on birth weight and gestational age.' *American Journal of Epidemiology 155*, 429–436.

Gordon, J. S. and Edwards, D. M. (2005) 'Mind body spirit medicine.' *Seminars in Oncology Nursing 21*, 3, 154–158.

Hatch, E. E. and Bracken, M. B. (1993) 'Association of delayed conception with caffeine consumption.' *American Journal of Epidemiology 138*, 12, 1082–1092.

Hinds, T. S. (1996) 'The effect of caffeine on pregnancy outcome variables.' *Nutrition Reviews 54*, 7, 203–207.

Laforenza, U., Patrini, C., Gastaldi, G. and Rindi, G. (1990) 'Effects of acute and chronic ethanol administration on thiamine metabolizing enzymes in some brain areas and in other organs of the rat.' *Alcohol and Alcoholism 25*, 591–603.

Leevy, C. M. and Baker, H. (1980) 'Vitamins and alcoholism.' *American Journal of Clinical Nutrition 21*, 1325–1328.

Maconochie, N., Doyle, P., Prior, S. and Simmons, R. (2007) 'Risk factors for first trimester miscarriage – Results from a UK-population-based case-control study.' *BJOG: An International Journal of Obstetrics & Gynaecology 114*, 170–186.

Mathews, F., Yudkin, P. and Neil, A. (1999) 'Influence of maternal nutrition on outcome of pregnancy: Prospective cohort study.' *British Medical Journal 319*, 339.

Milton, H., Erickson, E. L. and Rossi, S. I. (1976) *Hypnotic Realities: The Induction of Clinical Hypnosis and Forms of Indirect Suggestion.* Manchester, NH: Irvington Publishers.

Nykjaer, C., Alwan, N. A., Greenwood, D. C. *et al.* (2014) 'Maternal alcohol intake prior to and during pregnancy and risk of adverse birth outcomes: Evidence from a British cohort.' *Journal of Epidemiology & Community Health 68*, 6.

Odou, N. and Brinker, J. (2014) 'Self-compassion, a better alternative to rumination than distraction as a response to negative mood.' *The Journal of Positive Psychology, 10*, 5, 1–11.

Pert, C. (1999) *Molecules of Emotion: The Science behind Mind-Body Medicine.* New York: Simon & Schuster.

Sengpiel, V., Elind, E., Bacelis, J. *et al.* (2013) 'Maternal caffeine intake during pregnancy is associated with birth weight but not with gestational length: Results from a large prospective observational cohort study.' *BMC Medicine 11*, 42.

Sheng, C. (2001) 'Emerging paradigms in mind-body medicine.' *Journal of Alternative and Complementary Medicine 7*, 1, 83–91.

Upledger, J. (1997) *Your Inner Physician and You: Craniosacral Therapy and Somato Emotional Release.* Berkeley, CA: Atlantic Books.

Ventegodt, S., Thegler, S., Andreasen, T. *et al.* (2007) 'Clinical holistic medicine (mindful, short-term psychodynamic psychotherapy complemented with bodywork) in the treatment of experienced impaired sexual functioning.' *Scientific World Journal 7*, 324–329.

Energetic Qualities of Common Foods

A NOTE ON COOKING

As always, the particular qualities of a product will be affected by how it is processed and/or cooked.

Beef can be used as an example of this – a steak will nourish Qi and Blood (Yang and Yin) equally, and could be considered balanced in its energetic properties. If you fry this steak, you subject it to intense heat and increase the potential of Yang within it. The longer you cook the steak (well done as opposed to blue), the more potential of Yang and the less potential of Yin it contains; this needs to be borne in mind (see Appendix C).

A NOTE ON VITAMIN AND MINERAL CONTENT

I have not included the vitamin or mineral content of the various foods listed below, as to do so would take hundreds more pages. For more information, contact a practitioner of Chinese or naturopathic medicine.

ENERGETIC QUALITIES OF MEAT PRODUCTS

Food	Energetic qualities	Organs affected	Actions
Beef	Neutral and sweet.	Spleen and Stomach.	Qi and Blood tonic.
	Wild cattle such as buffalo can be included in this category. As is normally the case, wild animals will tend to be warmer (increased potential of Yang) in nature.		
Chicken	Warm and sweet.	Spleen and Stomach.	Qi tonic, warms the interior.
	Wild fowl such as pheasant can be included in this category. As is normally the case, wild animals will tend to be warmer (increased potential of Yang) in nature.		

cont.

Food	Energetic qualities	Organs affected	Actions
Duck	Neutral, sweet and salty.	Lung and Kidney.	Regulates the water Triple Burner, dispels oedema (Damp).
Goat	Warm, salty and slightly sweet.	Stomach, Spleen and Kidney.	Qi tonic.
Goose	Neutral, sweet and salty.	Lung and Stomach.	Lubricates dryness, regulates the water Triple Burner.
Ham	Warm and salty.	Spleen.	Qi tonic, produces Body Fluids, subdues rebellious Stomach Qi.
Lamb	Warm and sweet.	Spleen and Kidney.	Qi and Yang tonic, warms the interior.
	Wild sheep can be included in this category. As is normally the case, wild animals will tend to be warmer (increased potential of Yang) in nature.		
Pigeon	Warm and sweet.	Spleen and Stomach.	Qi tonic, treats chronic weakness.
Pork	Neutral, sweet and salty.	Spleen, Stomach and Kidney.	Lubricates dryness, tonifies Yin.
Rabbit	Sweet and slightly cool.	Liver and Large Intestine.	Stomach and Spleen Qi tonic.
Turkey	Warm and sweet.	Spleen and Stomach.	Qi tonic.
Venison	Warm, salty and slightly sweet.	Stomach, Spleen and Kidney.	Qi tonic.
	Wild venison will be hotter in nature.		
Eggs (Chicken)	Neutral and sweet.	Lung and Stomach.	Blood tonic, helps produce Body Fluids, lubricates dryness and dispels Empty Heat.

Egg white (Chicken)	Cool and sweet.	Lung.	Detoxifies and lubricates, clears Empty Heat, benefits the throat.
Egg yolk (Chicken)	Neutral and sweet.	Heart and Kidney.	Tonifies blood, lubricates dryness.
Eggshell	Cool and salty.	Stomach, Spleen and Liver.	Checks the production of excess gastric acid, arrests bleeding.

ENERGETIC QUALITIES OF FISH PRODUCTS AND SHELLFISH

Food	Energetic qualities	Organs affected	Actions
Oily fish	Cool and salty.	Lung, Stomach and Kidney.	Nourishes Yin, clears Heat.
White fish	Cool and salty.	Stomach, Lung and Kidney.	Blood tonic.
	Exceptions: Tuna, shark, sword fish and trout are all considered to be hot in nature and will therefore tonify Qi and Yang.		
Carp	Neutral and sweet.	Spleen, Stomach and Large Intestine.	Promotes lactation, heals swelling, guides downward, harmonises San Jiao.
Crab	Cold and salty.	Liver and Stomach.	Moves Blood, clears Heat.
Cuttlefish	Neutral and salty.	Liver and Kidney.	Liver Blood tonic, sharpens vision.
Mackerel	Sweet and salty.	Liver, Stomach and Kidney.	Yin and Blood tonic.
Mussels	Warm and salty.	Liver and Kidney.	Qi tonic, treats simple goitre due to Kidney Qi or Yang vacuity.

cont.

Food	Energetic qualities	Organs affected	Actions
Salmon	Neutral, sweet and salty.	Liver and Kidney.	Yin and Blood tonic.
Sea cucumber (sea ginseng)	Tonifies Yuan (original) Qi.	Kidney.	Tonifies the Kidney, treats chronic inflammation, strengthens the body.
Shrimp	Hot, sweet and salty.	Spleen and Kidney.	Tonifies Yang, dispels Cold in the interior.
Tuna	Warm and salty.	Spleen and Kidney.	Qi and Yang tonic.
Abalone	Neutral, sweet and salty.	Liver and Kidney.	Detoxifies the Liver, nourishes Liver Yin, sharpens vision.
Lobster	Warm, sweet and salty.	Spleen and Kidney.	Tonifies Qi, improves appetite.
Oysters	Neutral, sweet and salty.	Liver and Kidney.	Yin and Blood tonic.
Oyster shells	Cool and salty.	Heart, Liver and Kidney.	Stops sweating, astringes Jing, softens hardness.
Prawn	Warm and salty.	Spleen, Stomach and Kidney.	Qi and Yang tonic.

ENERGETIC QUALITIES OF DAIRY (COW) PRODUCTS

Food	Energetic qualities	Organs affected	Actions
Butter	Warm and sweet.	Lung and Stomach.	Qi and Blood tonic.
Cheese	Cool and sweet.	Lung and Large Intestine.	Lubricates the Lung and Large Intestine, quenches thirst, nourishes Yin.

Milk	Neutral and sweet.	Heart, Lung and Stomach.	Produces Body Fluids and lubricates the Intestines.

ENERGETIC QUALITIES OF COMMON VEGETABLES

Food	Energetic qualities	Organs affected	Actions
Aubergine	Cold and sweet.	Stomach and Large Intestine.	Clears Heat, cools Blood.
Beetroot	Neutral and sweet.	Heart and Spleen.	Builds Blood, guides downward.
Bell (sweet) pepper	Hot and pungent.	Heart and Spleen.	Warms the interior, harmonises the middle Jiao, stimulates appetite.
Broccoli	Cool and sweet.	Spleen.	Builds Blood.
Brussels sprouts	Warm and bitter.	Kidney and Spleen.	Tonifies Kidney and Spleen Qi.
Cabbage	Neutral and sweet.	Stomach and Large Intestine.	Promotes urination, clears Damp Heat in the Stomach and Intestines.
Carrot	Sweet and neutral.	Spleen, Liver and Lung.	Strengthens the Spleen, tonifies Liver Yin, clears Heat.
Cauliflower	Neutral and sweet.	Large Intestine.	Lubricates the Intestines.
Celeriac	Sweet and slightly warm.	Spleen and Kidney.	Dries Damp, promotes good digestion, tonifies Qi.

cont.

Food	Energetic qualities	Organs affected	Actions
Celery	Aromatic, sweet and cool.	Liver, Stomach and Bladder.	Clears Heat, sedates Liver fire, harmonises the Stomach, promotes urination.
Chard	Cool and sweet.	Stomach, Spleen, Large and Small Intestine.	Qi and Blood tonic, clears Heat, detoxifies, haemostatic.
Chicory/ endive	Bitter, sour and cool.	Liver and Gall Bladder.	Astringes Liver Blood.
Courgette (zucchini)	Cool and sweet.	Spleen and Kidney.	Nourishes Kidney Yin and Blood.
Cucumber	Cool and sweet.	Spleen, Stomach and Large Intestine.	Clears Heat, promotes urination, quenches thirst.
Fennel	Aromatic and warm.	Stomach, Kidney and Bladder.	Warms the interior, regulates the flow of Qi.
Jerusalem artichoke	Warm and sweet.	Spleen and Liver.	Dries Dampness, moves Liver Qi.
Kale	Warm and sweet.	Stomach and Spleen.	Tonifies Qi.
Kohlrabi	Warm and sweet.	Stomach and Spleen.	Dries Damp, moves Liver Qi.
Leek	Warm and aromatic.	Liver and Lung.	Qi and Yang tonic, regulates the smooth movement of Liver Qi, breaks Blood stasis, expels Cold from the interior.
Lettuce	Cool, bitter and sweet.	Stomach and Large Intestine.	Promotes urination, calms the mind.

Marrow	Cool and slightly sweet.	Stomach and Intestines.	Produces Body Fluids, nourishes Yin, lubricates the Intestines.
Melon	Cooling, sweet and slightly bitter.	Heart, Stomach and Kidney.	Cools Empty Heat in the Stomach, nourishes Kidney Yin.
Mustard greens	Warm and aromatic.	Lung, Spleen and San Jiao.	Dispels Phlegm and Damp, tonifies Spleen Qi.
Onion	Aromatic, warm and bitter.	Lung, Stomach and Large Intestine.	Tonifies Qi, dissolves masses (Qi and/or Phlegm stagnation), soothes the flow of Qi.
Parsnip	Warm and sweet.	Spleen and Lung.	Tonifies Qi and Blood, dries Damp.
Potato	Neutral and sweet.	Spleen, Stomach and Large Intestine.	Tonifies Spleen and Stomach Qi and Yin.
Pumpkin	Sweet and warm.	Spleen and Stomach.	Reinforces the middle Jiao, tonifies Qi.
Radish	Cold, pungent and sweet.	Lung and Stomach.	Detoxifies, promotes digestion, guides downward.
Spinach	Cool and sweet.	Large and Small Intestine.	Qi and Blood tonic, clears Heat, haemostatic, lubricates dryness.

cont.

Food	Energetic qualities	Organs affected	Actions
Spring onion (scallion)	Warm and pungent.	Lung and Stomach.	Raises Yang, tonifies and regulates Qi, dries Dampness, promotes urination, dispels Blood stasis, expels Cold from the interior.
Squash	Sweet and warm.	Stomach and Spleen.	Heals inflammation, relieves pain.
Swede	Sweet and slightly warm.	Stomach, Spleen and Lung.	Qi tonic, dries Damp, moves Qi.
Sweet potato	Neutral and sweet.	Stomach and Kidney.	Qi tonic.
Tomato	Cool, sweet and sour.	Stomach and Liver.	Clears Heat, produces Body Fluids, nourishes Yin.
Turnip	Cooling.	Liver and Spleen.	Diuretic, clears internal Heat, sharpens vision.

ENERGETIC QUALITIES OF COMMON GRAINS

Food	Energetic qualities	Organs affected	Actions
Amaranth	Slightly cool and sweet.	Stomach and Spleen.	Blood and Yin tonic.
Barley	Cool, sweet and salty.	Spleen and Stomach.	Harmonises Stomach Qi and promotes urination.
Buckwheat	Cool and sweet.	Large Intestine, Stomach and Spleen.	Blood tonic, dispels Empty Heat.

Flaxseed	Cool and slightly sour.	Liver and Stomach.	Nourishes Liver Yin and Blood.
Glutinous rice	Warm and sweet.	Spleen, Stomach and Lung.	Qi tonic.
Job's tears (adlay millet)	Cool and sweet.	Spleen, Lung and Kidney.	Spleen and Lung Qi tonic, diuretic.
Maize	Neutral, sweet and salty.	Heart and Kidney.	Tonifies Heart blood, calms the mind, drains Damp.
Malt	Warm and sweet.	Spleen and Stomach.	Promotes digestion.
Millet	Cool, sweet and salty.	Stomach, Spleen and Kidney.	Qi and Blood tonic, tonifies Yin, dispels Empty Heat, lubricates dryness, promotes proper digestive function.
Oats	Sweet and warm.	Heart and Spleen.	Qi and Blood tonic.
Quinoa	Neutral and warm.	Pericardium and Spleen.	Qi and Blood tonic.
Rice	Neutral and sweet.	Spleen and Stomach.	Spleen Qi tonic.
Rice bran	Neutral, sweet and pungent.	Stomach and Large Intestine.	Harmonises the Qi of the Stomach and Large Intestine and causes it to descend.
Rye	Neutral and bitter.	Spleen and Liver.	Dries dampness, diuretic.
Spelt	Neutral and cool.	Heart and Kidney.	Tonifies Heart and Kidney Yin.
Wheat	Cool and sweet.	Heart, Spleen and Kidney.	Astringes Heart Qi.
Wheat bran	Cool and sweet.	Stomach.	Cools Stomach fire.

cont.

ENERGETIC QUALITIES OF COOKING OILS

Food	Energetic qualities	Organs affected	Actions
Almond oil	Cool and sweet.	Lung, Spleen and Stomach.	Treats dry cough, nourishes Blood and Yin.
Avocado oil	Cool and slightly sweet.	Lung, Stomach and Large Intestine.	Cools and lubricates the Lung, moistens the Large Intestine, nourishes Yin.
Coconut oil	Warm, sweet and slightly aromatic.	Stomach and Large Intestine.	Produces Body Fluids, nourishes Blood and Yin.
Grapeseed oil	Neutral, slightly cool.	Liver and Stomach.	Tonifies Qi and Blood.
Olive oil	Neutral, sweet and sour.	Lung and Stomach.	Treats diarrhoea due to its obstructive nature.
Peanut oil	Neutral and sweet.	Spleen and Lung.	Lubricates the Lung, harmonises the Stomach.
Rapeseed oil	Neutral.	Spleen and Kidney.	Treats post-partum pain due to wind invasion.
Sesame oil	Cool and sweet.	Lung and Large Intestine.	Detoxifies, lubricates dryness in the Large Intestine.
Sunflower oil	Neutral, slightly warm and sweet.	Stomach and Lung.	Moistens the Lung and Intestines, tonifies Blood.
Walnut oil	Warm and sweet.	Spleen and Kidney.	Warms the Spleen and Kidney Qi.

Animal oils

Butter	Warm and sweet.	Lung and Stomach.	Qi and Blood tonic.
Lard	Warm and sweet.	Lung, Stomach and Spleen.	Moistens dryness, lubricates the intestines, nourishes Blood and Yin.

ENERGETIC QUALITIES OF COMMON SWEETENERS

Food	Energetic qualities	Organs affected	Actions
Brown sugar (cane sugar)	Cold and sweet.	Lung and Stomach.	Produces Body Fluids, promotes urination, guides obstruction downward.
Honey	Neutral and sweet.	Lung, Spleen and Large Intestine.	Detoxifies, lubricates dryness.
Molasses	Sweet and slightly warm.	Spleen and Large Intestine.	Nourishes Blood and Yin.
White sugar	Neutral and sweet.	Spleen.	Produces Body Fluids, lubricates the Lung.

ENERGETIC QUALITIES OF COMMON KITCHEN HERBS AND SPICES

Food	Energetic qualities	Organs affected	Actions
Alfalfa (sprouts)	Cool and slightly bitter.	Heart and Bladder.	Clears Heat in the Bladder, calms the mind.
Angelica	Warm and sweet.	Lung, Stomach and Large Intestine.	Builds Blood and nourishes Yin.

cont.

Food	Energetic qualities	Organs affected	Actions
Anise	Warm, aromatic and sweet.	Spleen, Liver and Kidney.	Qi tonic, expels Cold from the body.
Bamboo shoots	Cold and sweet.	Stomach.	Clears Stomach Heat; cook with meat to moderate its heating effects.
Basil	Warm and aromatic.	Lung, Spleen, Stomach and Large Intestine.	Qi tonic, moves Blood, improves digestive function.
Borage	Cool.	Lung and Stomach.	Nourishes Lung Yin.
Caraway	Warm and slightly aromatic.	Kidney and Stomach.	Warms and harmonises Stomach, moves Qi in the middle Jiao.
Chamomile	Neutral.	Heart, Stomach, Spleen and Large Intestine.	Calms the mind, harmonises the digestive system.
Chilli pepper (hot)	Warm and sweet.	Spleen and Stomach.	Qi tonic, dries Damp, moves Qi and Blood.
Chives	Warm and aromatic.	Liver, Stomach and Kidney.	Qi tonic, moves Qi and Blood.
Cinnamon (bark)	Warm and aromatic.	Kidney, Spleen and Bladder.	Qi tonic, warms the interior.
Cloves	Warm and aromatic	Spleen, Stomach and Kidney.	Tonifies Spleen and Kidney Qi, moves Blood.
Coriander	Warm and aromatic.	Heart and Spleen.	Reduces abdominal swelling, promotes digestive function, promotes sweating.

Cumin	Neutral and slightly cool.	Stomach and Liver.	Moves Qi in the middle Jiao, improves digestive function.
Curry leaf	Warm, aromatic and slightly bitter.	Stomach, Spleen and Large Intestine.	Qi tonic, dries up Damp, warms and tonifies the Qi of the Large Intestine.
Dill	Warm and aromatic.	Kidney, Spleen and Lung.	Warms the Stomach and Spleen, tonifies Kidney Qi.
Fennel	Warm and aromatic.	Kidney, Bladder and Stomach.	Warms the lower Jiao, tonifies Bladder and Kidney Qi, guides out food stagnation.
Fenugreek	Warm, aromatic and slightly sour.	Kidney.	Tonifies Kidney Qi.
Galangal	Warm and aromatic.	Stomach and Lung.	Dries Damp, tonifies Qi.
Garlic	Warm and aromatic.	Lung, Spleen and Stomach.	Qi tonic, dries Dampness, kills worms.
Ginger	Warm and aromatic.	Spleen and Lung.	Dries Damp, tonifies Qi, subdues rebellious Stomach Qi.
Hops	Cool and bitter.	Heart and Stomach.	Calms the mind, harmonises the Stomach.
Horseradish	Warm, aromatic and slightly bitter.	Lung and Spleen.	Qi tonic, dries Dampness.
Juniper	Warm and aromatic.	Kidney and Spleen.	Dries Dampness, tonifies Qi.
Lavender	Aromatic, bitter and slightly sweet.	Heart.	Calms the mind, nourishes Heart Yin.

cont.

Food	Energetic qualities	Organs affected	Actions
Lemon balm	Aromatic and cooling.	Lung and Stomach.	Clears Wind Heat.
Liquorice	Neutral and sweet.	All Zang and Fu.	Harmonises the entire body, counteracts toxins, calms the Stomach.
Marjoram	Aromatic and cold.	Heart, Pericardium and Stomach.	Clears Wind Heat, induces sweating.
Marshmallow	Cool, slightly sweet and slightly sour.	Stomach and Kidney.	Produces Body Fluids, lubricates the Intestines.
Mint	Aromatic, cold and slightly sour.	Lung, Stomach and Liver.	Clears Wind Heat, moves Liver Qi, harmonises the digestive system.
Nutmeg	Warm and aromatic.	Spleen and Large Intestine.	Qi tonic, causes Qi to descend.
Oregano	Aromatic and warm.	Lung and Spleen.	Clears Wind Cold, induces sweating, warms the Spleen.
Paprika	Warm, sweet and slightly bitter.	Heart and Spleen.	Tonifies Heart and Spleen Blood.
Parsley	Cool and slightly bitter.	Heart and Bladder.	Tonifies Blood, clears Heat in the Bladder.
Peppermint	Aromatic and cool.	Lung and Liver.	Treats skin rashes caused by Heat, moves Liver Qi.
Rosemary	Warm and pungent.	Lung.	Induces sweating, moves Qi.
Saffron	Neutral and sweet.	Heart and Liver.	Qi and Blood.

Sage	Aromatic and warm.	Lung and Stomach.	Moves Qi in the chest, harmonises the digestive organs.
Star anise	Aromatic, warm and sweet.	Spleen, Liver and Kidney.	Tonifies Qi (especially defensive Qi), moves Qi.
Stinging nettle	Cool and sour.	Liver and Kidney.	Tonifies Liver Yin and Blood tonic.
Szechuan peppercorn	Warm and aromatic.	Spleen, Large Intestine and Kidney.	Qi tonic, Qi mover, warms the middle and lower Jiao.
Tarragon	Warm, aromatic and bitter.	Lung, Spleen and Kidney.	Qi tonic, moves Qi, dries Damp.
Thyme	Neutral and aromatic.	Lung.	Stops cough, opens the chest, dries Damp.
Turmeric	Warm and aromatic.	Liver.	Moves stagnant Qi, reduces swelling.
Vanilla	Warm and sweet.	Spleen.	Harmonises the digestive system.
Vinegar	Warm, sour and bitter.	Liver and Stomach.	Detoxifies, stops bleeding.
Watercress	Aromatic and cool.	Lung and Stomach.	Clears Wind Heat and Stomach Heat.

ENERGETIC QUALITIES OF COMMON FRUITS

Food	Energetic qualities	Organs affected	Actions
Apple	Cool, sweet and sour.	Liver and Lung.	Promotes digestion, clears Liver Heat, lubricates the Lung.

cont.

Food	Energetic qualities	Organs affected	Actions
Apricot	Neutral, sweet and sour.	Lung and Large Intestine.	Stops cough, produces Body Fluids, lubricates the Large Intestine.
Avocado	Cool and sweet.	Stomach and Large Intestine.	Lubricates the Intestines, builds Body Fluids.
Banana	Cold and sweet.	Spleen, Stomach and Intestines.	Lubricates the Intestines, detoxifies, clears Heat.
Blackberry	Sour and slightly sweet.	Liver, Kidney and Bladder.	Astringes Liver Blood and Jing, tonifies the Bladder Qi.
Blackcurrant	Sweet and slightly cool.	Stomach and Spleen.	Builds Blood, nourishes Yin.
Blueberry	Cooling and sour.	Kidney and Liver.	Tonifies Liver and Kidney Yin.
Cherry	Warm and sweet.	Spleen and Kidney.	Treats cold-type rheumatism (Bi Syndrome), numbness due to Blood vacuity.
Coconut	Warm and sweet.	Stomach and Spleen.	Produces Body Fluids, nourishes Yin and Blood, promotes urination.
Cranberry	Cooling and sour.	Heart, Bladder and Liver.	Clears Heat in the Bladder, dispels vacuous Heart Heat, astringes Liver Blood.
Fig	Neutral and sweet.	Spleen and Large Intestine.	Treats constipation, vacuity diarrhoea, haemorrhoids.

Gooseberry	Sour and slightly cold.	Liver.	Moves stagnant Liver Qi, good to treat digestive upsets caused by Qi stagnation.
Grape	Neutral, sweet and sour.	Lung, Spleen and Kidney.	Qi and Blood tonic, strengthens tendons and bones, promotes urination.
Grapefruit	Aromatic, cold, sweet and sour.	Spleen and Stomach.	Treats indigestion due to rebellious Stomach Qi, good to promote appetite.
Lemon	Sour and astringent.	Spleen and Liver.	Treats invasion of Summer Heat, quietens a restless foetus.
Lime	Aromatic, sour and astringent.	Spleen and Liver.	Supports prolapse, clears Phlegm.
Mulberry	Cooling.	Heart, Stomach, Liver and Kidney.	Reduces fever, quenches thirst, clears Heat in the Small Intestine, promotes Blood circulation.
Orange	Cold and damp.	Spleen, Stomach and Lung.	Clears internal Heat, guides Stomach downward, produces Body Fluids.
Orange peel	Warm and aromatic.	Spleen, Stomach and Lung.	Moves stagnant Qi, dries up Damp, expels Wind Cold.
Peach	Warm, sweet and sour.	Lung, Liver and Stomach.	Lubricates the Intestines, promotes Blood circulation, produces Body Fluids.

cont.

Food	Energetic qualities	Organs affected	Actions
Pear	Cooling, sweet and slightly sour.	Lung and Stomach.	Treats Lung or Stomach Yin deficiency, lubricates dryness in the Lung or Large Intestine.
Pineapple	Neutral, sweet and sour.	Lung, Stomach and Bladder.	Quenches thirst, promotes urination, heals inflammation.
Plum	Neutral, sweet and sour.	Liver and Kidney.	Produces Body Fluids, promotes urination.
Pomegranate	Cool and sweet.	Lung and Stomach.	Produces Body Fluids, quenches thirst.
Quince	Cool and sour.	Liver and Kidney.	Moves Liver Qi, invigorates Qi and Blood circulation in the legs.
Raspberry	Warm, sweet and sour.	Liver and Kidney.	Astringes Liver Blood and Kidney Jing, tones the Bladder.
Redcurrant	Sour and cold.	Heart and Liver.	Astringes Heart and Liver Blood, builds Body Fluids.
Strawberry	Cool, sweet and sour.	Heart, Pericardium, Lung and Stomach.	Clears Heat, produces Body Fluids, moistens the Lung.
Watermelon	Cold and sweet.	Heart, Stomach and Bladder.	Clears Heat, promotes urination, lubricates the Intestines.

REFERENCES AND FURTHER READING

Benskey, D. (1993) *Chinese Herbal Medicine: Materia Medica*. Vista, CA: Eastland Press Inc.

Lu, H. C. (2002) *Chinese Natural Cures: Traditional Methods for Remedy and Prevention*. New York: Black Dog & Leventhal Publishers, Inc.

Ni, M. (2009) *Tao of Nutrition*. Ashland, OH: SevenStar Communications.

Pitchford, P. (2002) *Healing with Whole Foods: Asian Traditions and Modern Nutrition*. Berkeley, CA: North Atlantic Books.

Wood, R. (1999) *The New Whole Foods Encyclopedia: A Comprehensive Resource for Healthy Eating*. Harmondsworth: Penguin Books.

Therapeutic Actions of Vitamins and Minerals

Clive McKay, a nutritional therapist working in the 1930s, estimated that in order to keep up with the published literature on nutrition, you would need to read one article every three minutes every working day. (And this would only have covered the chemical aspects of food, ignoring the medical implications.)

There are four things to be aware of before you take nutritional supplements:

- Always bear in mind that excessive quantities of vitamins or minerals can be toxic in nature, and while trying to address any perceived imbalances, always take only the recommended daily dosage. If you are unsure of what you need, seek professional advice.

- When purchasing vitamin or mineral supplements, opt for high-quality chelated products made from natural substances rather than synthetic compounds produced in a laboratory.

- Take a moment to evaluate the health of your digestive system. Poor digestive function with the resultant symptoms of chronic tiredness, low energy, poor muscle tone, etc. are common reasons why people take nutritional supplements. A digestive system that can't absorb nutrients from food will likely not be able to break down and assimilate nutrients in supplement form either. If you recognise these symptoms in yourself, try a very bland, totally cooked diet for two weeks. If energy levels improve and there are less symptoms of digestive issues such as bloating after eating, begin taking your supplements again. The chances are that your digestive system will have recovered sufficiently to assimilate the nutrients that they contain.

- Liquid supplements, either shop-bought or homemade in the form of stocks and stews, are also an excellent way to improve the chances of assimilating nutrients. The work of digestion is done in the cooking pot, thus relieving pressure on an overburdened digestive system. It should be noted that cooking tends to have a negative impact on the vitamin (B vitamins especially) content of food. Adding miso paste at the end of cooking can help redress this issue.

- The best way of addressing imbalances is via a good diet, assuming your digestive system is functioning properly (see above).

SUPPLEMENTAL USE OF MINERALS IN NATUROPATHIC AND CHINESE MEDICINE

Boron

Essential for: Healthy bones and joints.

Deficiency: May lead to osteoporosis and arthritis.

Food sources: Fruits and vegetables.

Therapeutic uses of supplements: To treat osteoporosis and arthritis.

Uses in Chinese medicine: Jing tonic, clears toxic Heat.

Calcium

Essential for: Healthy bones and teeth, muscle contraction, a healthy heart and nervous system, blood pressure regulation and blood clotting.

Deficiency: Leads to nerve and bone disorders, osteoporosis, high blood pressure and pre-eclampsia of pregnancy, and may contribute to colon cancer.

Food sources: Leafy green vegetables.

Therapeutic uses of supplements: To treat osteoporosis, high blood pressure, tooth problems, muscle cramps, pre-eclampsia and heart disease.

Uses in Chinese medicine: Tonifies Kidney Yin and calms the mind.

Chloride

Chloride is the main negative charged electrolyte (anion) found outside of the body's cells. It controls fluid and electrolyte balance when combined with sodium and potassium.

Essential for: Maintaining a normal fluid balance within the body's cells and tissues.

Deficiency: Rare.

Food sources: Found in heavy doses in salt.

Uses in Chinese medicine: Tonifies Kidney Yin and Jing. Calms the mind.

Chromium

Essential for: Normal sugar and fat metabolism because it is part of a compound known as glucose tolerance factor (GTF).

Deficiency: Symptoms include high blood fat and cholesterol levels, glucose intolerance and other diabetes-like symptoms. Marginal deficiency may play a role in the development of diabetes and heart disease.

Food sources: Liver, eggs, poultry and whole grain cereals. The chromium content of food varies with the location in which the food is grown.

Uses in Chinese medicine: Spleen Qi tonic.

Cobalt

Cobalt is a component of vitamin B12. The average body content of cobalt is less than 1 mg and it is stored in the muscles, bone, liver and kidneys.

Essential for: The only known role of cobalt is as part of the vitamin B12 molecule. Many of the functions of vitamin B12 are mediated through the cobalt portion of the molecule. This includes the synthesis of DNA, production of red blood cells, maintenance of nerve function, and absorption and metabolism of nutrients.

Deficiency: Equivalent to a deficiency of vitamin B12, with symptoms of pernicious anaemia, nerve disorders and abnormalities in cell formation. However, these symptoms cannot be treated with cobalt alone.

Food sources: Green leafy vegetables, some fish, liver, kidney and milk.

Therapeutic uses of supplements: There are no uses for cobalt supplements. Radioactive cobalt-60 is used to treat some cancers.

Uses in Chinese medicine: Qi tonic, expels worms.

Copper

Essential for: Normal metabolism, healthy bones, joints, skin and blood vessels, a healthy nervous system, a healthy cardiovascular system, the formation of haemoglobin in red blood cells, a healthy immune system, and absorption and metabolism of nutrients.

Deficiency: Leads to anaemia, connective tissue defects, immune suppression, nerve problems and heart disease.

Food sources: Seafood, meat and whole grains.

Therapeutic uses of supplements: Used to treat heart disease and arthritis.

Uses in Chinese medicine: Tonifies Spleen Qi and dispels Dampness.

Iodine

Essential for: Normal metabolism, growth and development as it is a component of thyroid hormones.

Deficiency: Leads to hypothyroidism, goitre and cretinism, and may play a role in fibrocystic breast disease.

Food sources: Vegetables grown in iodine-rich soil, iodised salt, seafood and milk. The iodine content of food varies with the location in which the food is grown.

Therapeutic uses of supplements: Used to treat deficiency disorders and also to treat fibrocystic breast disease. Topical iodine is used as an antiseptic.

Uses in Chinese medicine: Builds Liver and Kidney Yin.

Iron

Essential for: The main element in the production of haemoglobin. Also needed for many other enzymes that are essential to our survival.

Deficiency: Vitamin C helps the absorption of iron; therefore deficiency of vitamin C may cause iron deficiency.

Food sources: Whole grains, vegetables, meat and eggs.

Uses in Chinese medicine: Yin and Blood tonic.

Magnesium

Essential for: Production and transfer of energy, a healthy heart, bones, muscles and blood vessels, protein and carbohydrate metabolism, transport of substances across cell membranes and manufacture of genetic material

Deficiency: Symptoms include fatigue, and mental and heart problems. Marginal deficiency may lead to cardiovascular disease, hypertension, diabetes, osteoporosis, asthma, migraine, premenstrual syndrome (PMS) and kidney stones.

Food sources: Whole grains, nuts and green vegetables.

Therapeutic uses of supplements: Treatment of stress, fatigue, cardio-vascular disease, migraine, kidney stones, asthma, PMS, osteo-porosis, muscle cramps, pre-eclampsia and diabetes.

Uses in Chinese medicine: Moves Qi and calms the mind.

Manganese

Essential for: Energy production, the action of the antioxidant enzyme, protein metabolism, bone formation and a healthy nervous system.

Deficiency: Rare. Marginal deficiency may play a role in osteoporosis and diabetes.

Food sources: Nuts, whole grains, dark green leafy vegetables and black teas. The manganese content of food varies with the location in which the food is grown.

Therapeutic uses of supplements: Used to treat inflammatory conditions, fatigue, mental disorders, epilepsy and diabetes.

Uses in Chinese medicine: Nourishes Kidney Yin.

Molybdenum

Essential for: Reactions involving the waste products of protein metabolism, iron utilisation, carbohydrate metabolism and alcohol and sulphate detoxification.

Deficiency: Rare and only seen in people who are on long-term tube or intravenous feeding or who have a rare genetic inability to use molybdenum. Symptoms include rapid heartbeat and breathing, headache, night blindness, anaemia, mental disturbance, nausea and vomiting.

Food sources: Milk, kidney, soya and beans, bread, liver and cereals. The molybdenum content of food varies with the location in which the food is grown.

Therapeutic uses of supplements: Used to detoxify copper in cases where levels are too high.

Uses in Chinese medicine: Tonifies Blood and Yin, clears Blood Heat.

Nickel

Nickel may be an essential trace mineral but its role in the body is unknown. The average adult body contains about 10 mg of nickel and it is found in many body tissues.

Essential for: High concentrations of nickel are found in genetic material and it may be involved in protein structure and function. It may also play a role in hormone function, and may activate certain enzymes related to the breakdown or utilisation of glucose.

Deficiency: Nickel deficiency in animals leads to decreased growth, dermatitis, pigment changes, liver damage and reproductive abnormalities. No deficiency symptoms have been reported in humans. Low blood levels of nickel may be found in those with liver and kidney disease.

Food sources: Vegetables usually contain more nickel than other foods. High levels have been found in cruciferous vegetables (cabbage family), spinach, lettuce and nuts.

Uses in Chinese medicine: Tonifies Kidney Yin.

Phosphorus

Essential for: Healthy bones, acid base balance in the body, metabolism of proteins, carbohydrates, fats and DNA, and energy production and exchange.

Deficiency: Rare; symptoms include weakness, loss of appetite, bone pain, joint stiffness, irritability, numbness, speech disorders, tremor and mental confusion.

Food sources: Meat, wheat germ, poultry, cheese, milk, canned fish, nuts and cereals. The functions of calcium, magnesium and phosphorus are closely related, and disturbances in one mineral may affect the other.

Therapeutic uses of supplements: Rare, but used to treat bone problems including osteomalacia, osteoporosis and rickets.

Uses in Chinese medicine: Tonifies Kidney Yin and Jing.

Potassium

Essential for: Water balance in the body, muscle contraction, acid–alkali balance, nerve impulse transmission, energy metabolism, protein and carbohydrate metabolism, and a healthy heart and blood vessels.

Deficiency: May lead to an increased risk of high blood pressure.

Food sources: Fruit, vegetables and whole grains.

Therapeutic uses of supplements: Used to treat cases of depletion, fatigue, high blood pressure, cardiovascular disease and kidney stones.

Uses in Chinese medicine: Drains Dampness.

Selenium

Essential for: The function of the antioxidant enzyme, glutathione peroxidase, which protects against damage to cells, healthy immune and cardiovascular systems, and hormone production.

Deficiency: May contribute to cancer, heart disease, arthritis, cataracts, autoimmune diseases and birth defects.

Food sources: Organ meats and seafood. The selenium content of food varies with the location in which the food is grown.

Therapeutic uses of supplements: May be useful in preventing heart disease, cancer and cataracts, and in the treatment of asthma and rheumatoid arthritis.

Uses in Chinese medicine: Tonifies Yin and calms the mind.

Silicon

Silicon, the most abundant mineral in the earth's crust, may be an essential element in humans. It is present in bone, blood vessels, cartilage, tendons, skin and hair.

Essential for: Silicon is found in areas of active growth inside bones and may be involved in the growth of bone crystals and calcification. Silicon may also play a role in the formation of cartilage and other connective tissue, giving strength and stability. It may help to maintain the elasticity of arterial cell walls.

Deficiency: Silicon deficiency in animals causes weak and malformed bones of the arms, legs and head. Low silicon levels also lead to atherosclerotic lesions in animals due to its role in artery wall formation. Thus silicon deficiency may play a role in cardiovascular disease.

Food sources: Silicon is widely available in food. Good sources include wheat, oats, rice, lettuce, cucumbers, avocados, parsnips and strawberries. Silicon is easily lost in food processing, however.

Therapeutic uses of supplements: Used to improve strength in hair, skin and nails. Silicon may have a role in the prevention and treatment of osteoporosis as supplements have been shown to increase bone mineral density.

Uses in Chinese medicine: Liver Yin and Blood tonic.

Sodium

Essential for: Water balance in the body, muscle contraction, acid–alkali balance nerve impulse transmission, energy production and stomach acid production.

Deficiency: Rare, and toxic effects from high intakes are of greater concern. Deficiency may occur in high temperatures due to hard exercise or manual work.

Food sources: Processed meats, cheese and butter.

Therapeutic uses of supplements: Usually unnecessary and an acquired taste. Sodium bicarbonate may be used to treat metabolic and respiratory acidosis.

Uses in Chinese medicine: Tonifies the Kidneys and Liver. Softens hardness.

Sulphur

As a constituent of all proteins, sulphur is an essential element for humans. The sulphur content of the average adult body is approximately 100 mg and most of this occurs in the three amino acids cysteine, cystine and methionine. The rest is in the form of sulphates attached to other substances in body cells.

Essential for: Sulphur is found mainly in tissues that contain high amounts of protein. It is a constituent of collagen, the protein found in connective tissue, bones and teeth; and keratin, the protein found in skin, hair and nails. Sulphur gives these tissues strength, shape and hardness. Sulphur is involved in the formation of bile acids which are important for fat digestion and absorption. As a component of the B vitamins thiamin and biotin, sulphur helps in the conversion of proteins, carbohydrates and fats to energy. Sulphur plays a part in the reactions that help cells utilise oxygen. It is necessary for blood clotting and for the function of several enzymes including glutathione and coenzyme A, and for the production of the hormone insulin.

Deficiency: No known sulphur deficiency disease. Protein is the main dietary source and a diet inadequate in protein would be of greater concern.

Food sources: Mustard, egg, seafood, beans, milk, milk products, nuts and meat. Protein supplies most of the sulphur in the diet but some comes in the form of sulphates in water, fruit and vegetables.

Therapeutic uses of supplements: As a mild laxative; a mild antiseptic in ointment form to treat acne, eczema, dermatitis and psoriasis; a parasiticide in lotion form to treat scabies; and as a depilatory agent. Oral sulphur has been used to treat psoriasis. Bathing in water containing sulphur may benefit arthritis sufferers.

Uses in Chinese medicine: Clears Heat toxin (infection).

Vanadium

Vanadium is a trace mineral that has been considered essential for humans since the 1970s. Vanadium is found in the blood, organ tissues and bones.

Essential for: Vanadium may act as a co-factor for enzymes involved in blood sugar metabolism, lipid and cholesterol metabolism, bone and tooth development, fertility, thyroid function, hormone production and neurotransmitter metabolism.

Deficiency: Not been described in man. Deficiency in animals causes infertility; a reduction in red blood cell production leading to anaemia; iron metabolism defects; and poor bone, tooth and cartilage formation. It is possible that deficiency in humans may lead to high cholesterol and triglyceride levels and increase susceptibility to heart disease and cancer.

Food sources: Whole grain breads and cereals, vegetable oils, nuts, root vegetables, parsley, fish, radishes, dill, lettuce and strawberries. The vanadium content of food depends on the soil in which it is grown.

Therapeutic uses of supplements: Animal experiments have shown that vanadium can mimic the effects of insulin and reduce blood sugar levels from high to normal. Vanadium supplements have been used as performance enhancers by athletes, although there is little research evidence to support their effectiveness.

Uses in Chinese medicine: Harmonises the Triple Burner.

Zinc

Essential for: Energy production, manufacture of genetic material, detoxification of chemicals, including alcohol, healthy immune and reproductive systems, hormone production, normal growth and development, and healthy brain, teeth, bones and skin.

Deficiency: Symptoms include skin problems, foetal abnormalities, reproductive defects, cardiovascular disease, immune deficiency, loss of eye function and osteoporosis.

Food sources: Seafood, meat and whole grains.

Therapeutic uses of supplements: Often given to diabetics and pregnant women. Also used to treat immune deficiency, the common cold, skin disorders, infertility, arthritis, taste disorders, macular degeneration, digestive diseases, prostate problems and to promote wound-healing.

Uses in Chinese medicine: Tonifies Jing.

SUPPLEMENTAL USE OF VITAMINS IN NATUROPATHIC AND CHINESE MEDICINE

Vitamin A: Retinol

Essential for: Healthy eyes and vision, growth, repair and cell differentiation, health of epithelial cells, protection against infection, and a healthy reproductive system.

Deficiency: Symptoms include night blindness, xerophthalmia, dry skin, retarded growth and increased susceptibility to infection and cancer.

Food sources: Liver, butter, whole milk and egg yolks.

Uses in Chinese medicine: Tonifies Blood and Yin, dispels Blood Heat.

Vitamin B1: Thiamin

Essential for: Releasing energy from food, carbohydrate and fatty acid metabolism, healthy growth, healthy skin, blood, hair and muscles, a healthy brain and nervous system, and alcohol metabolism.

Deficiency: Symptoms include fatigue, depression, reduced mental functioning, muscle cramps, nausea, heart enlargement and eventually beriberi, which can cause paralysis. Alcoholics are at particular risk of thiamin deficiency.

Food sources: Meat, whole grains, fish and nuts.

Uses in Chinese medicine: Qi tonic.

Vitamin B2: Riboflavin

Essential for: The production of energy from food, normal growth and development, a healthy immune system, healthy skin, hair and blood cells, iron, pyridoxine and niacin functions, hormone function and a healthy nervous system and brain.

Deficiency: Symptoms include red, swollen, cracked mouth and tongue; fatigue; depression; anaemia; and greasy, scaly skin on the face, body and limbs. Deficiency may also contribute to cataract formation.

Food sources: Meat, dairy products and fortified grains.

Uses in Chinese medicine: Lung Qi tonic.

Vitamin B3: Niacin

Essential for: The release of energy from food, healthy skin, blood cells and digestive system, normal growth and development, hormone production, a healthy brain and nervous system, and repair of genetic material.

Deficiency: Eventually leads to pellagra, with symptoms of dermatitis on the hands and face, weakness, appetite loss, sore mouth, diarrhoea, anxiety, depression and dementia.

Food sources: Meat, fish, pulses and whole grains.

Uses in Chinese medicine: Qi tonic.

Vitamin B5: Pantothenic acid

Essential for: The release of energy from food, cholesterol and fatty acid metabolism, healthy red blood cells, a healthy immune system, healthy adrenal gland function and a healthy nervous system.

Deficiency: Rare in humans except in cases of general malnutrition. Symptoms in animals include greying of hair, decreased growth and adrenal gland abnormalities.

Food sources: Yeast, liver, eggs, wheat germ, milk, meat, poultry and whole grains. It is also produced by bacteria in the gut.

Uses in Chinese medicine: Can help clear Damp Heat from the Liver and Gall Bladder Channels (jaundice).

Vitamin B6: Pyridoxine

Essential for: Pyridoxine co-enzymes function at all levels of the metabolism of proteins, amino acids, production of haemoglobin and in new proteins being produced by the body. It is also an essential nutrient needed to produce glycogen phosphorylase which breaks down muscle glycogen for fuel.

Deficiency: Chronic low-grade inflammation, depression (low energy, feeling down) and mental confusion.

Food sources: Wheat germ, chicken, fish and eggs.

Uses in Chinese medicine: Qi tonic (Spleen Qi).

Vitamin B12: Cyanocobalamin

Essential for: Energy release from food, amino acid and fatty acid metabolism, healthy nerves, blood cells, skin and hair, production of genetic material, and growth and development.

Deficiency: Leads to pernicious anaemia with symptoms of fatigue, lightheadedness, headache and irritability. Other symptoms include nausea, loss of appetite, sore mouth, diarrhoea, abnormal gait, loss of sensation in hands and feet, confusion, memory loss and depression.

Food sources: Meat, fish, eggs and dairy products.

Uses in Chinese medicine: Qi tonic.

Vitamin C: Ascorbic acid

Essential for: The manufacture of collagen, a protein that forms the basis of connective tissues such as bones, teeth and cartilage, wound-healing, healthy immune and nervous systems, adrenal hormone production and as an antioxidant.

Deficiency: Severe deficiency leads to scurvy with symptoms of bleeding gums, joint pain, easy bruising, dry skin, fluid retention, and depression. Marginal deficiencies may play a role in the development of cancer, cardiovascular disease, high blood pressure, lowered immunity, diabetes and cataracts.

Food sources: Fruit and vegetables.

Uses in Chinese medicine: Clears Heat, benefits the defensive Qi.

Vitamin D: Cholecalciferol

Essential for: The absorption and use of calcium and phosphorus, which are vital for functions such as the development of bones and teeth, healthy nervous and immune systems, regulation of some hormones, and normal cell growth and maturation.

Deficiency: Deficiency in children leads to rickets in which bones lose calcium and become soft and curved. In adults, symptoms include bone pain and tenderness, and muscle weakness. Deficiency may also increase the risk of osteoporosis, arthritis and cancer.

Food sources: Oily fish, liver and eggs.

Uses in Chinese medicine: Jing and Yin tonic.

Vitamin E: Alpha tocopherol

Essential for: Its action as an antioxidant to provide protection for cells against free radical damage which may lead to disorders such as heart disease and cancer. It is particularly important in protecting fats, cell membranes, DNA and enzymes against damage.

Deficiency: Rare. Symptoms in infants include irritability, fluid retention and anaemia; and in adults, lethargy, loss of balance and anaemia. Marginal deficiencies may increase the risk of heart disease, cancer and premature ageing.

Food sources: Wheat germ, nuts and seeds, whole grain cereals, eggs and leafy greens.

Uses in Chinese medicine: Blood mover.

Vitamin K: Phylloquinone

Essential for: Blood clotting, bone metabolism and kidney function.

Deficiency: Deficiency in adults is rare and is usually limited to those who have liver or food absorption disorders. Symptoms include prolonged clotting time, easy bleeding and bruising. It may contribute to osteoporosis. Deficiency can occur in premature babies.

Food sources: Dark leafy greens, oils from green plants and some dairy products. Vitamin K is also produced by gut bacteria.

Uses in Chinese medicine: Tonifies the Large Intestine and Lung Qi and Spleen Blood.

Folate: Folic acid

Essential for: The synthesis of genetic material, protein metabolism, healthy pregnancy, healthy red blood cells, bones and hair, and healthy nervous, digestive and immune systems.

Deficiency: Symptoms include anaemia, mood disorders and gastrointestinal disorders. Deficiency in pregnancy causes neural tube defects in babies. Low levels may increase the risk of heart disease and cancer.

Food sources: Liver, pulses and dark green leafy vegetables. Caution: High intake levels of folate may mask the test for some diseases (pernicious anaemia being the most common).

Uses in Chinese medicine: Qi and Jing tonic.

OTHER COMMON NUTRITIONAL SUPPLEMENTS
THAT ARE THERAPEUTICALLY USEFUL
Coenzyme Q10: Ubiquinone

Essential for: Energy production, ATP formation and antioxidant action.

Deficiency: Affects the heart. It has also been linked to other conditions such as cancer, muscular dystrophy, diabetes, obesity, periodontal disease, lowered immune function and neurodegenerative disorders such as Parkinson's disease.

Food sources: Found in all plant and animal foods. Good sources include meat, fish and vegetable oils.

Therapeutic uses of supplements: Used to treat cardiovascular disease, cancer, high blood pressure, periodontal disease and muscular dystrophy. Coenzyme Q10 may also be useful in preventing the side effects of beta blockers and statin-type cholesterol-lowering drugs. In Japan Coenzyme Q10 has been used successfully to treat hundreds of thousands of heart patients.

Uses in Chinese medicine: Harmonises San Jiao.

Essential fatty acids

Essential for: Normal nerve function and reducing inflammation.

Deficiency: Dry skin, dandruff, brittle nails, constipation, aching joints, premenstrual syndrome (PMS) and depression.

Food sources: Oily fish, grass-fed beef, nuts and seeds.

Therapeutic uses of supplements: Treatment of inflammatory conditions such as arthritis and hormone balance. Some studies have linked regular consumption of essential fatty acids to a reduction in cognitive disorders such as dementia.

Uses in Chinese medicine: Liver and Kidney Yin tonic, harmonises the Triple Warmer.

Glucosamine

Essential for: Making glycosaminoglycans, proteins that are the key structural components of cartilage. Glucosamine also stimulates the cells that produce these structural proteins and helps to normalise cartilage metabolism by inhibiting breakdown and exerting anti-inflammatory effects.

Food sources: None.

Therapeutic uses of supplements: Used to help the body to repair damaged or eroded cartilage and has been used to treat osteoarthritis. Short-term human trials suggest that glucosamine sulphate may produce a gradual and progressive reduction in joint pain and tenderness, as well as improved range of motion and walking speed. Results of the trials have also shown that glucosamine has produced consistent benefits in patients with osteoarthritis and that, in some cases, it may be equal or superior to anti-inflammatory drugs in controlling symptoms. It is often combined with chondroitin, a substance that has anti-inflammatory properties and protects the cartilage against breakdown. It has also been used to promote wound-healing and to treat psoriasis (see Braun and Cohen 2015).

Uses in Chinese medicine: Tonifies Liver and Kidney Yin.

REFERENCES AND FURTHER READING

Aguilaniu, H., Durieux, J. and Dillin, A. (2005) 'Metabolism, ubiquinone synthesis, and longevity.' *Genes & Development 19*, 20, 2399–2406.

Ballentine, R. (2005) *Diet and Nutrition: A Holistic Approach*. Honesdale, PA: Himalayan Institute Press.

Brandt, K. D. (1987) 'Effects of nonsteroidal anti-inflammatory drugs on chondrocyte metabolism in vitro and in vivo.' *American Journal of Medicine 83*, suppl. 5A, 29–34.

Braun, L. and Cohen, M. (2015) *Herbs and Natural Supplements, Volume 2* (4th edn). Australia: Churchill Livingstone.

Crolle, G. and D'Este, E. (1980) 'Glucosamine sulfate for the management of arthorosis: A controlled clinical investigation.' *Current Medical Research and Opinion 7*, 105–109.

Holick, M. F. (2005) 'Vitamin D: Important for prevention of osteoporosis, cardiovascular heart disease, type 1 diabetes, autoimmune diseases, and some cancers.' *The Southern Medical Journal 98*, 10, 1024–1027.

Palan, P. R., Connell, K., Ramirez, E. *et al* (2005) 'Effects of menopause and hormone replacement therapy on serum levels of coenzyme Q10 and other lipidsoluble antioxidants.' *Biofactors 25*, 1–4, 61–66.

Pitchford, P. (2002) *Healing with Whole Foods: Asian Traditions and Modern Nutrition*. Berkeley, CA: North Atlantic Books.

Shield, M. J. (1993) 'Anti-inflammatory drugs and their effects on cartilage synthesis and renal function.' *European Journal of Rheumatology and Inflammation 13*, 7–16.

Wesseling-Perry, K. and Salusky, I. B. (2009) 'Is replacement therapy with nutritional and active forms of vitamin D required in chronic kidney disease mineral and bone disorder?' *Current Opinion in Nephrology and Hypertension 18*, 4, 308–314.

Wood, R. (1999) *The New Whole Foods Encyclopedia: A Comprehensive Resource for Healthy Eating*. Harmondsworth: Penguin Books.

Cooking Methods

Casseroles: The casserole is similar to soups and stews but casseroling tends to be a warmer cooking method. The long oven cooking in direct heat infuses fire energy (Yang Qi) deeply into the food, and this method is especially good for people sensitive to cold or in cold weather.

Roasting: This is a very warming method of cooking that is ideal for winter and for those with a cold constitution.

Salads: Raw food is generally cleansing and cooling, and suits those with an excess and Hot constitution. In the Western culture of excess, some salad is helpful provided the digestive system is strong enough to cope with it. However, raw food fads do not work well in a climate that is too cold and damp to tolerate the over-consumption of raw foods.

Soups and stews: These have the benefit of releasing nutrients easily and so are particularly helpful for those with weak digestive systems. They are unlikely to congest the digestive system because all the ingredients are broken down by the cooking process.

Steaming and boiling: These are considered fairly neutral methods of cooking that do not significantly increase a food's energetic temperature but nevertheless help release nourishment easily to our bodies. Steamed food tends to be mildly cleansing, and steaming is generally a better, more gentle option for those seeking the radical cleansing effects of the raw food diet.

Stir fry: This classic oriental method is now popular in the West. This is a tasty and nourishing method, a little warmer than steaming. It is also very quick, which has obvious appeal in the fast-track Western world. Adding ginger and garlic or other warming spices helps make the food warmer and often easier to digest.

Glossary of Terms

Amenorrhoea: The absence of a menstrual period in a woman of reproductive age.

Anovulation: A menstrual cycle during which the ovaries do not release an egg.

Basal body temperature (BBT): The lowest body temperature attained during rest (usually during sleep). It can be used as a baseline while tracking hormonal changes.

Blastocyst: In humans, blastocyst formation begins about five days after fertilisation. It has a diameter of about 0.1–0.2 mm and comprises 200–300 cells.

Blood: A Yin substance that has cooling, moistening and nourishing functions.

Blood deficiency: A lack of Blood.

Clomiphene citrate (Clomid): A medication prescribed to induce ovulation.

Cold: A term that can be used to describe the decreased functioning of a Zang or Fu, or impediment of the free flow of one or more of the Five Vital Substances caused by a lack of Qi or Yang. Cold is present in biomedical hypo conditions such as hypoadrenalism, hypoglycaemia or hypothyroidism.

Damp Heat: A condition of Dampness and Heat combined (typical in inflammatory conditions).

Dampness: An accumulation of fluids within an area of the body or within the body generally.

Decoction: A combination of herbs that is cooked or brewed to make a soup or medicinal tea.

Deficiency: An insufficiency of Qi, Blood, Yin, Yang or Essence.

Diuretic: A medicinal substance that rids the body of excess fluid, usually by promoting urination.

Dryness: An external pathogenic factor (EPF) or a condition resulting from Blood or Yin deficiency.

Dysmenorrhoea: Pain during menstruation.

Ectopic pregnancy: A complication of pregnancy in which the embryo attaches outside the uterus.

Eight Principles: Four sets of factors used by practitioners of Chinese medicine as a starting point in diagnosis. The Eight Principles are represented by internal/external, cold/heat, excess/deficiency and Yin/Yang.

Empty Heat: A deficiency of Yin, leading to heat symptoms of a transient nature. Empty Heat can also be caused by a lack of free movement. There will be heat, inflammation and fever, but it is all just a result of stagnation; as soon as free flow is restored, the heat disappears. Try this experiment: cut some grass and make a pile out of it; take the temperature in the centre of the pile. Leave the grass to sit for a day and take the temperature again – the temperature will have gone up because it is fermenting (stagnating). The same thing occurs inside a human body, causing the illusion of heat.

Endometriosis: A condition in which tissue that normally grows inside the uterus grows outside it.

Endometrium: The inner mucous membrane of the uterus.

Essence (Jing): A fluid substance that is the material basis of all organic life. It acts as a blueprint governing the unfoldment of all organic processes at various stages of life. Issues governed by conception and pregnancy are typically treated via Essence (and Kidneys).

Excess: Can be viewed as too much, too prolonged, inappropriate or in the wrong context.

Excess Yang: Excess heat, a condition of True Heat.

Excess Yin: Excess cold, a condition of True Cold.

External: Pathogenic factors that attack the body from the exterior.

Fallopian tubes: Two very fine tubes leading from the ovaries into the uterus.

Fibrocystic breast disease: This is a condition where one or both breasts become tender, painful and lumpy. The roundish lumps can be soft or firm, move freely within the breast tissue and are tender to the touch. The intensity of symptoms may vary with the menstrual cycle.

Fire: Extreme Heat.

Five Phases: The five energies of Wood, Earth, Metal, Water and Fire.

Follicle-stimulating hormone (FSH): Secreted by the pituitary gland, and regulates the development, growth and reproductive processes of the body.

Gestational diabetes: Occurs when women who have never had diabetes before develop an impaired ability to process glucose during pregnancy, resulting in high blood sugar.

Gonadotropin-releasing hormone (GnRH) agonist: A synthetic amino acid that interacts with the gonadotropin-releasing hormone receptor to elicit the release of the pituitary hormone's follicle-stimulating hormone (FSH) and luteinising hormone (LH).

Human chorionic gonadotropin (hCG): A hormone produced by the embryo after implantation.

Hypothalamus: One of the most important functions of the hypothalamus is to link the nervous system to the endocrine system via the pituitary gland. The hypothalamic–pituitary–ovarian axis is a critical part in the development and regulation of the reproductive system.

Internal: Pathologies that originate in or affect the inside of the body.

Intracytoplasmic sperm injection (ICSI): An in vitro fertilisation procedure in which a single sperm is injected directly into an egg.

Laparoscopy: An operation performed in the abdomen or pelvis through small incisions with the aid of a camera. It can either be used to inspect and diagnose a condition or to perform surgery.

Luteinising hormone (LH): A hormone produced by the pituitary gland. An acute rise of LH (LH surge) triggers ovulation.

Menopause: The time in a woman's life when menstrual periods stop permanently, and they are no longer able to have children.

Meridians (Channels): The pathways through which the Five Vital Substances flow.

Non-steroidal anti-inflammatory drugs (NSAIDs): A class of drugs that provide pain-killing (analgesic), fever-reducing (antipyretic) and anti-inflammatory effects.

Oestrogen: The primary female sex hormone, responsible for the development and regulation of the female reproductive system and secondary sexual characteristics.

Oligomenorrhoea: Menstrual periods occurring at intervals of greater than 35 days, with only four to nine periods in a year.

Organs: *See Zang Fu.*

Ovarian cyst: A fluid-filled sac within the ovary.

Ovulation: The release of an egg from the ovaries.

Pelvic inflammatory disease (PID): An infection of the upper part of the female reproductive system – the uterus, fallopian tubes and ovaries – and the inside of the pelvis.

Pituitary gland: Hormones secreted from the pituitary gland help control thyroid function as well as certain aspects of sexual function and the normal development of a growing foetus.

Polycystic ovary syndrome (PCOS): A set of symptoms due to elevated levels of male hormones (androgens) in women.

Progesterone: Prepares the uterus for implantation and then helps maintain pregnancy.

Prostaglandins: A group of lipid (fats and fat-soluble vitamins) compounds that have hormone-like effects.

Qi: The vital energy that flows through the Channels (Meridians).

Qi deficiency: A lack of Qi.

Qi Gong: A set of exercises used to move and regulate the Five Vital Substances.

Seven Emotions: Sadness, fright, fear, grief, anger, joy and pensiveness. Any one of these emotions experienced in excess can be considered as potential causes of illness.

Shen: The spirit and mental faculties of a person.

Six External Evils: Wind, Cold, Summer Heat, Dampness, Dryness and Fire.

Stagnation: A blockage that prevents the free flow of one or more of the Five Vital Substances.

Summer Heat: An external pathogenic factor (EPF).

Tai Chi Chuan: A set of exercises used to move and regulate the Five Vital Substances.

Tao: The ancient philosophy of oneness in all creation.

Tonification/tonify: To nourish, support or strengthen.

Toxicity: Inflammation, such as that manifested in infection.

Triple Burner or Triple Warmer: The three production centres for energy and water.

Tuina: A traditional Chinese massage technique that focuses on Channels and acupoints rather than the musculature of the body, as in Western massage.

Wei Qi: Defensive energy; it acts like the immune system in biomedicine.

Wind: An external pathogenic factor (EPF).

Yang: Heat and the body's ability to generate and maintain warmth and circulation.

Yang deficiency: A cold condition in which there is a lack of Yang (movement and warmth).

Yin: The ability to cool and moisten.

Yin deficiency: A lack of cooling and moistening that results in Heat.

Zang Fu: The functional aspects of organs.

Index